YOUR FIRST PREGNANCY

An Essential Guide

70000040490

KT-431-712

£8.99

WITHDRAWN FROM STOCK

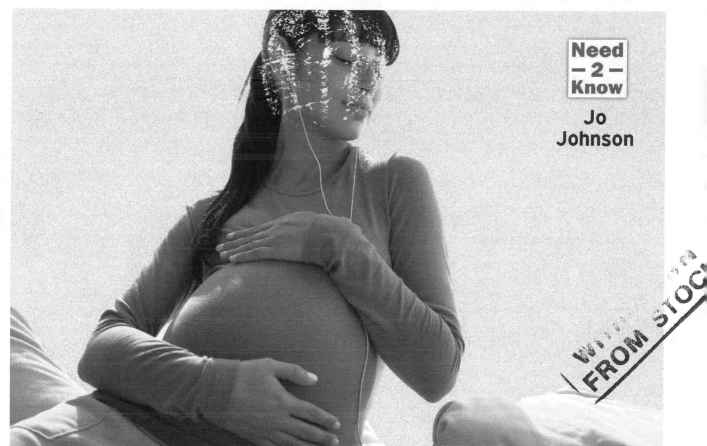

Need
— 2 —
Know

Jo
Johnson

First published in Great Britain in 2009 by
Need2Know
Remus House
Coltsfoot Drive
Peterborough
PE2 9JX
Telephone 01733 898103
Fax 01733 313524
www.need2knowbooks.co.uk

Need2Know is an imprint of Forward Press Ltd.
www.forwardpress.co.uk
All Rights Reserved
© Jo Johnson 2009
SB ISBN 978-1-86144-066-2
Cover photograph: Jupiter Images

T000000 40490

Contents

WITHDRAWN FROM STOCK

Introduction

Finding out you are pregnant is a life-changing event, whether it is a surprise or something you have been planning. Giving birth dates back to the start of life on earth but hasn't become any less daunting or worrying over the years.

Some women find they embrace the experience and enjoy every last minute of bringing a new life into the world, while others find they are uncertain throughout; both are totally normal and are experienced by women all over the world.

The information found in this book will help ease your fears, answer all your questions and guide you through your first pregnancy. As the title suggests, it will equip you with all the information you'll need: from practical issues like when to try for a baby and how to deal with an unexpected pregnancy to coping with the physical changes to your body and preparing for the birth. With separate chapters dedicated to the expectant father and those who find out they are having more than one baby, you'll find everything you need to know.

By the end of the book you will have gained a sound knowledge of the physical side of pregnancy, how your emotions will change, how you will cope and what to expect in the future. Having this information will leave you free to relax, enjoy your pregnancy and look forward to meeting your new arrival.

Disclaimer

This book is for general information about pregnancy and is not intended to replace professional medical advice. It can be used alongside medical advice, but anyone planning a pregnancy or with concerns about their pregnancy is strongly advised to consult their healthcare professional.

National recommendations can change, so it is important to consult your healthcare professional before acting on any of the information in this book.

WITHDRAWN FROM STOCK

Chapter One

Family Planning – Your Pre-pregnancy Plan

Congratulations on deciding to start your family. You are about to embark on a remarkable journey filled with anticipation and joy.

The decision to start a family is a big one, so by making sure you are prepared you will find the experience that little bit less stressful and altogether more enjoyable.

Is it the right time?

Is there ever a right time to start a family? For some people, it is part of their life plan and something that has been scheduled to fit in with their lifestyle and career. For others, it just happens unexpectedly but is often the best surprise they have ever had.

Many couples want to make sure they are married and have a home of their own before they enhance their life with a child. Others are less organised but know that a child can easily fit in with their existing circumstances.

It doesn't really matter whether your pregnancy has been planned or if it was a surprise. As long as you are ready to make the changes necessary to ensure the best of health for you and your baby, you can enjoy your pregnancy.

'The decision to start a family is a big one, so by making sure you are prepared you will find the experience that little bit less stressful and altogether more enjoyable.'

Your relationship

In an ideal world everyone would pick the perfect partner to have a child with. For a lot of people, this does happen. Unfortunately, for some women their choice of partner is fine while in a sexual relationship but when a child joins the equation the partner finds he is not ready.

If you are in a committed relationship, the subject of whether you are going to have a family one day is something that probably should be addressed to make sure you both want the same things out of life. Having a child can stress even the most solid of relationships, so it really is in your best interests to find out what your partner's opinions on children are. This way, you can decide whether he is the best person to be the father of your child.

You may want to discuss how your relationship will change after a child has been born, how you will organise your working lives, your plans for the future and what rules you will introduce with regard to social lives and discipline. Some families never discuss these issues and they don't ever present a problem, while other people will admit that it would have been useful to set some ground rules before a pregnancy was conceived.

On the other hand, there are many women who decide that they can shoulder parenthood alone and seek donor insemination from a fertility clinic. These women are often financially, emotionally and spiritually sound and are able to cope with lone parenting.

'In an ideal world money shouldn't be an issue with regard to having a child but realistically it is something that can affect your life dramatically.'

Careers and finance

In an ideal world money shouldn't be an issue with regard to having a child but realistically it is something that can affect your life dramatically.

Are you ready for the financial sacrifices you will have to make when your child is born? Newborn babies don't really need a lot in the first few months but equipment such as Moses' baskets, cots, pushchairs and car seats will require some initial outlay. Many couples are fortunate enough to have friends and relatives who pass on or buy these items, but if you don't have this luxury you may need to save up. Try to remember that babies have no style or fashion sense and aren't aware of not having items at the top of the range. As most items are only used for the first few years, buying the most expensive is not necessary and a cheaper alternative will do just as well.

With regard to your career, you may want to consider whether you are where you want to be or whether you want to spend a few more years climbing the career ladder. It can be very difficult to do training, go on courses or work full time when you have a young child, despite the best efforts of your employer and the government.

Spend some time thinking about what hours you want to do when you return to work after having a baby and whether your current job will fit in with family life. You may need to re-assess your working situation. You might decide that you want to stay at home while your child is in the pre-school years. There are many options available to you and now is the time to start thinking about your long term career and family life.

Emotional issues

Being a mother is not a job, it's a way of life. You are planning to share your life with someone that you don't yet know and this can be a very daunting prospect. However, it is good that you are taking the issue seriously, giving it some real thought and spending some time reading up on the subject.

Pregnancy can affect your emotional state because of the changes to your body, the impending responsibility and your changing hormone levels. To be a good parent all you need to do is prepare to be a good role model and know that you have enough love to share. Your child will rely on you for everything in the first few months and during this time you are likely to be tired and exhausted, despite your best efforts to uphold the idealistic images of pregnancy and childbirth that we are bombarded with. As long as you are confident in your capability to love your child, and are happy that the child's father or your partner is comfortable with their new role, you will probably be just fine.

If you have had a history of emotional issues or depression, please see your doctor so they can monitor your welfare and plan any interventions that you may need in the future.

Home environment

When you are planning a child you may want to pay some attention to your home environment. For example, a violent or abusive environment is not going to promote a healthy upbringing for any child. If you have concerns, spend some time thinking about what changes you can make to create a more secure and loving environment.

With regard to location, some couples like to plan ahead and move to somewhere that is in the catchment area of the school they would like their child to go to. Unfortunately, the choice of schooling for children is not as wide as it used to be and this can influence where some families decide to live.

Is your home heated? Does it need any work doing to make it safe for a child? Do you have access to hot water? These may be basic questions but with more and more people finding it harder to juggle their finances, they are issues that many people have to address before considering a pregnancy.

Some homes have animals that may not be suitable to keep with young children. For example, some dogs adopted from rescue centres aren't safe with young children. This may not have been a problem before but may be something that needs to be considered now.

Lifestyle factors

Making sure your body is healthy and ready for pregnancy is one of the greatest advantages you can give to your future child. Your lifestyle significantly impacts on the health of your potential child and there are steps you can take to make sure your body is ready for the miraculous journey that is about to take place.

Diet

Your diet is extremely important when you are hoping to become pregnant. Eating healthily will benefit both you and your potential or existing baby.

In the weeks before you are aiming to conceive, you should be taking a folic acid supplement on top of eating a healthy diet. Folic acid is part of the vitamin B group of nutrients and plays a major role in the health of a developing foetus. Although it is found in many food sources such as kale and spinach, it can be difficult to get the recommended 400mg every day. All women who are thinking of having a baby or who are in the early stages of pregnancy should be taking a supplement.

A lack of folic acid can lead to births defects including those of the brain and spinal cord. These parts of the foetus develop very early on which is why women should be taking the supplement before they become pregnant to ensure their body already has a supply. It is recommended that the supplement is taken until at least week 12 of the pregnancy. If you are planning to conceive, swap the time you normally take your contraceptive pill for the folic acid supplement. By doing this, you should never forget to take it.

As your blood supply is going to increase, you should make sure you are getting enough iron from your diet as this is vital for the production of red blood cells. Green vegetables, red meat and bread are all good sources of iron, but there are also many products that are now fortified with iron, making it even easier to ensure you have a good supply.

Protein and carbohydrates are both essential parts of a healthy diet as they provide the building blocks for cell and bone production and give energy respectively. Lean fish, meat, fruit, vegetables, pulses and breads will give you all you need to keep yourself and the foetus healthy.

Many companies make supplements especially for those hoping to become pregnant or those who are already expecting. Although these may be beneficial to some women, they are in no way meant to replace a healthy diet that contains all the required food groups. It is also not recommended that you follow a specific diet or weight loss plan while you are pregnant unless it is under the guidance and advice of your doctor or midwife.

Foods to be wary of and limit excessive consumption of include products high in vitamin A (e.g. oily fish) as these can be detrimental to the health of your foetus, raw fish and meat as these increase the chances of food poisoning and any type of pâté as it can contain listeria.

'In the weeks before you are aiming to conceive, take a folic acid supplement on top of eating a healthy diet.'

When you are trying for a baby and throughout any pregnancy, make sure you drink plenty of water or fruit juice to keep your cells hydrated. As your blood volume increases and your baby grows, you will need extra fluids to make sure you are healthy, along with the increased fluids needed for breast milk production. Small amounts taken more often will encourage a healthy pregnancy.

Exercise

Getting in shape is a great idea when you are planning a pregnancy. Not only will your body cope better with the changes, but you will increase the oxygen levels in your body which you will pass on to your baby while it is developing.

Try and exercise about three times a week in order to gain the most benefits.

If you think you may already be pregnant and participate in contact sports or heavy weight lifting, you may want to think about amending the sport to suit your circumstance or changing the type of activity you do as you could be endangering your pregnancy.

'Try and exercise about three times a week in order to gain the most benefits.'

As your pregnancy progresses, you may find that you need to swap the exercise you do to something gentler, such as swimming or yoga. There are many classes that are geared specifically towards pregnant women and contain exercises that are designed for your changing circumstance and shape.

Tobacco and alcohol

If you are a smoker then there is no better time to give your body the break it needs and quit. Even one cigarette can harm an unborn child. In men, tobacco can decrease fertility by negatively affecting the quality of sperm.

Low birth weight and the increased chance of having a stillbirth or a premature delivery are just some of the dangers that you are risking by smoking. Every cigarette is filled with poisons and, in effect, a smoking mother is knowingly harming her child. Even those with a 'light' cigarette habit are risking the life of their child.

Try and imagine how difficult it is to continue smoking when you are looking after a baby. You can't smoke indoors and you can't leave a baby alone to go outside. By giving up now, you are significantly improving the chances of having a healthy baby and maintaining your own health and ability to care for it. This is without mentioning the financial implications that smoking can bring.

Speak to your doctor about joining a support group or finding out about nicotine replacement therapy before you try and conceive. Quitting before you get pregnant will give your body the best chance of carrying a healthy baby.

The role of alcohol while pregnant has caused some confusion over the past few years, and experts are still trying to determine whether drinking alcohol is safe during pregnancy. The general advice is that sticking to the recommended one unit a day will not pose any threat to your baby. Some people argue that it may actually be beneficial, however this does not mean that non-drinkers should suddenly start drinking.

If you are not yet pregnant and are not driving after drinking, there is no reason why you can't continue to have a glass of wine in the evening or as you normally would.

For more information on safe alcohol consumption, visit the Department of Health website at www.dh.gov.uk.

Sex

Many men and women worry about having sex when they are trying for a baby and when a pregnancy has occurred. There is no need to worry as sex is a healthy activity and will do absolutely nothing to harm the unborn child.

When you are planning to conceive, it is recommended that you have sex around your most fertile time. A woman ovulates 14 days before her next period is due and this is when you should be trying.

Over the years there have been conflicting opinions about the frequency of sex and whether it improves the chances of becoming pregnant or not. In theory, the more sex you have, the higher your chances of becoming pregnant. However, most doctors agree that having sex more than once a day may decrease the quality and strength of the sperm. There is also a train of thought that suggests that the longer a man goes without an ejaculation, the less motility the sperm has. This means it may lack the strength and speed needed to reach the fallopian tubes and meet an egg ready for fertilisation.

Given all the information available, you can be safe in the knowledge that you are more likely to conceive if you enjoy sex around the time of ovulation and a few days either side.

Try not to worry too much about the right time to conceive as the stress and rigidity this can bring may actually lower your chances of success. If you are concerned that you are not getting your timing right, there are ovulation prediction kits available to buy that can help you determine the exact date of your ovulation.

When you are having sex, try and let gravity help nature along by finding a position that encourages the sperm to remain inside the vagina for a little while. It is also advantageous to avoid anal sex as the chances of transferring unhealthy bacteria from the anus to the vagina are high. If an infection develops, it can hinder your chances of conceiving.

Ceasing contraception

No matter how long you have been using contraception for or what type you have been taking, the effects are reversible. When you stop using them, your fertility is most likely to be restored to the same degree as it was before.

When to stop using contraception

Contraception may be stopped at any time. You don't have to take your pill, use your diaphragm, cap or condoms as long as you are confident that you or your partner is not carrying any sexually transmitted infections, or you are aware of your infection status.

If, however, you are using the hormone implant or injection or have been fitted with an intra-uterine coil device, more simply known as an IUD (though this is unusual in people who have not had any children yet), you will need to see your doctor and let its effects wear off before you can conceive.

If you cease using any form of the pill, condom or female condom, your fertility will be restored almost immediately and conception may occur during your next sexual encounter.

Learning about your cycle

Health professionals agree that it is in the woman's best interests to have at least one regular cycle between ceasing contraception and conceiving. The bleed experienced when using hormone-based contraception is not a true period and exists only as a way of reassuring the user that she is not pregnant (however, it must be remembered that the bleed does not actually prove this medically).

If you are planning to start your family, it can be beneficial to have a regular cycle or two as a way of determining when your most fertile time is. This can be achieved by learning how many days there are in your cycle and figuring out when you are ovulating (releasing an egg).

A normal female cycle may have as little as 21 days between each bleed or up to 35 days or more. It doesn't matter how long your cycle is as long as it is normal for you.

When am I most fertile?

If you have a regular cycle, it is fairly easy to work out when you are ovulating and are at your most fertile. Technically, a female is fertile from the time she starts her periods until they end during the menopause. Of course, this doesn't suggest that either end of this spectrum should be promoted as the right time, but biologically it is possible.

When you are thinking of starting your family, spend a few months jotting down exactly when you start and stop bleeding and how many days there are between each bleed. You will ovulate exactly 14 days before your next period, so it is most advantageous to have unprotected sex around this time. Fertilisation may not occur immediately after sex as sperm can live in the female body for around 72 hours after ejaculation.

'Technically, a female is fertile from the time she starts her periods until they end during the menopause. Of course, this doesn't suggest that either end of this spectrum should be promoted as the right time.'

There are also predictor kits available to buy in the chemist or the supermarket but these can be costly, so be prepared for the charges. However, they are very useful for women who don't have regular cycles.

Some women say that they can feel ovulation take place by experiencing a heightened sex drive and a raised body temperature during this time.

If you are still having trouble, please see your GP who will be able to give you more advice and help you decide when you are most likely to conceive.

Conceiving while using contraception

Many women worry when they find out they are pregnant and realise they have been using contraception. The most common worry surrounds using hormone-based contraceptives such as the pill, the implant or the injection.

Scientists have found that there is very little or no detrimental effect to either the developing foetus or the mother when this has occurred. If you are taking the pill and think you may be pregnant, it is worthwhile taking a pregnancy test to determine whether conception has occurred before you stop taking the pill. Obviously, the sooner you do this the better, as you can take steps to make sure you are in optimal health for your pregnancy. If you are sure you are pregnant, stop taking the pill today.

It has also been found that using these types of contraception makes no difference to the result of a pregnancy test despite them both being hormone-based. The type of hormone that is produced when you are pregnant is different to that contained in hormone-based contraceptives.

Making sure you are free from disease

If you are planning a family and have been sexually active in the past, it may be beneficial to tell your doctor of your plans and that you want to make sure you are free from any diseases (especially sexually transmitted infections) before you stop using contraception, especially condoms.

Both you and your partner may want to be tested if you feel there is any risk of either of you carrying any diseases or infections.

During this time your doctor may also carry out a few basic tests to check your overall health and make sure your body is in a good enough condition to carry a healthy pregnancy.

Summing Up

Whether you suddenly find yourself expecting or have been planning a baby for some time, it is never too late to start taking care of yourself and planning for the future. Having a baby is one of life's most important decisions and shouldn't be taken lightly. There are many things to consider when you are trying to conceive or are pregnant already. Your diet, lifestyle and general health may play a great role in how easy your pregnancy is, your own health in the future and how fit and well your baby grows while in the womb and after.

Making a few simple changes today could allow you to reap many benefits later in life and may ensure you give birth to a healthy baby.

Chapter Two

Discovering You Are Pregnant

Whether you have planned it or not, finding out you are pregnant can stir up some very strong emotions ranging from surprise, shock and panic to elation, contentment and excitement. This experience will be totally individual to you and no one can guess how you will feel. You may take it all in your stride or you may find you need a few days to get used to the idea.

Some women have no idea they are pregnant until the doctor tells them or they take a test, as they don't experience any of the common symptoms. Others find that they have all the usual ones and some that are pretty unique too!

The give-away signs of pregnancy

Not all women have the luxury of planning exactly when they are going to start their family, and some do not realise they are expecting until well into the pregnancy or, very rarely, until labour starts. But there are some signs and symptoms that indicate you are in the early stages and can lead you to take a pregnancy test.

Missing a period

Missing a period is the most common sign of pregnancy. It can, however, be confused by teenage girls for delayed puberty or a settling-in time while their cycle regulates itself. Women approaching the menopausal years may

'This experience will be totally individual to you and no one can guess how you will feel.'

confuse the changes for part of the menopausal process. Unless these women experience other signs, they may not suspect they are pregnant until they are quite a way in.

A period may be delayed or missed entirely, thus indicating a pregnancy. Perhaps you are just a few days late and are a little curious as to why, or maybe you have just realised that you haven't had a period at all this month. Whether your period is just a little late or has been missed altogether, you should take a pregnancy test to either confirm or rule out a pregnancy.

Missing a period isn't the only sign of pregnancy, so it is helpful to have an understanding of the other common signs just in case.

Spotting

Some women find that they have had a period but it was a little lighter or different to their usual monthly bleed. This can be spotting, in which case there is a bleed but it normally only lasts a few days and is a lot lighter than a normal period.

'Missing a period is the most common sign of pregnancy.'

Spotting occurs as the fertilised egg implants into the wall of the womb and grows into an embryo. As the implantation occurs, the wall can bleed a little and this is what can be confusing. This spotting normally only lasts for the first month and can cause the woman to delay taking a test as they believe it to be their normal period.

If there is a possibility that you are pregnant and have not taken a test, and you are experiencing spotting or bleeding accompanied by pain in the lower abdomen, seek medical advice immediately as this can be a sign of an ectopic pregnancy which will need urgent medical attention.

Breast changes

As your breasts prepare to feed a baby, the tissues must change to accommodate the demand that may be put on them. This can cause either pain or soreness, though some women may find they do not experience any breast changes at all.

The breast tissue and glands within the breast are changing and developing very quickly during this time and may change in size and shape even during the early weeks. This is very normal and shows that a healthy pregnancy is occurring.

Soreness

Breast soreness can range from slight tenderness and discomfort to acute pain that can bring you to tears. Some women find that even the lightest touch or smallest amount of friction from very basic activities such as going up and down the stairs can cause quite severe pain. On the other hand, some women state that they feel a little uncomfortable but it's nothing unmanageable.

Pain and discomfort may be eased by changing the type of bra you are wearing to something soft and supportive. A sports bra is usually very good at relieving some of the discomfort, though it is not worthwhile buying an expensive one as you will probably need to buy a larger size as your pregnancy continues. You may not fit into it again even after the birth of your baby.

Nipple changes

Many women are surprised to learn how much their nipples change in the early weeks of pregnancy. The area around the nipple itself is called the areola, and this can grow larger in size and deepen in colour. You may also find that you grow a few nipple hairs during your pregnancy as a result of changing hormone levels, but this is nothing to worry about and demonstrates a healthy pregnancy. That said, if you don't experience any changes to your nipples, this doesn't mean that your pregnancy is not progressing as normal.

If you find small pale lumps around the areola, do not worry as these are also part of the pregnancy. They are known as Montgomery's tubercules and are not a sign of something serious.

The nipple itself may also grow larger and more prominent, again this is nothing to be worried about. In fact, this may help you breastfeed your baby in the future. All of these changes should subside in the months following the birth of your baby, however your breasts themselves may not return to the exact condition or appearance they were previously in, even if you don't breastfeed.

Nausea and vomiting

The term 'morning sickness' is a frequently used phrase, even by medical professionals sometimes, but it is a little misleading. This experience will be totally individual to you and no one can guess how you will feel. Some women find they are sick at the same time every day while others may only suffer from an occasional bout of nausea. Some women do not experience any sickness at all.

There are several remedies available for easing these symptoms, with ginger being one of the oldest and most reliable. Take regular fluids and try nibbling ginger biscuits as a way of staving off nausea.

Nausea and vomiting can be signs of other physical conditions, so if you cannot keep any food in your system or the vomiting is making you feel weak, speak to your doctor.

'This experience will be totally individual to you and no one can guess how you will feel.'

Cravings

Cravings are not experienced by all women and are often over-exaggerated in films and books, as most cravings are for very mundane types of food or drink. However, there are some women who find they are yearning for some very strange concoctions.

For the most part, cravings are harmless and do not usually last for the entire pregnancy. Some of the weirder cravings can be damaging to health as women have reported that they longed for the smell of petrol, paint, ashtrays and even glue, all of which should never be inhaled. If you are struggling to control a potentially harmful craving, speak to your doctor or midwife as they may be able to help you.

Some women feel deprived of a very important part of pregnancy if they do not have any cravings, but it is common to have none at all. Just think how many calories you are saving yourself by not having any chocolate cravings, and how much nutritional benefit you can provide to your baby while you are in total control of your diet.

Tiredness and lethargy

Tiredness is a common part of being pregnant but something that most people do not associate with the early signs of discovering a pregnancy. Obviously, tiredness can occur as a result of lifestyle, stress or illness, and should be assessed by your doctor if it continues for several weeks and pregnancy has been ruled out.

As your body changes and your energy supplies are busy developing your baby, you may find you are struggling to get through the day and wonder how you'll cope when you have a baby. Don't worry, this tiredness does not last and should subside shortly after the first three months, leaving you filled with a new zest for life.

Try to get an extra hour or two of sleep at night and eat small but regular meals during the day to keep your energy levels up. It may also be helpful to avoid fluids after the early evening as you will be less likely to get up to go to the toilet during the night. However, you must make sure you are taking plenty of fluids during the day.

'Try and get an extra hour or two of sleep at night and eat small but regular meals during the day to keep your energy levels up.'

Heightened senses

Finding you have a heightened sense of smell, and therefore taste, is another common indication that you are expecting. Scientists think this may be because of hormonal changes in the body and that oestrogen, the female sex hormone, is to blame.

All of a sudden you may discover smells and aromas in your normal surroundings that you hadn't even noticed before. This isn't a problem for some women, but others can be repelled by what are otherwise quite normal smells.

If preparing the evening meal is turning you off, why not just have sandwiches for tea? There is no rule that you must have a hot meal every day, and often sandwiches can be more filling and nutritious and a lot quicker to prepare. Alternatively, ask your partner or friends to cook, or treat yourself to a meal out.

Your sense of smell should return to normal after the pregnancy and you will probably be a lot more tolerant of the aromas that repel you at this time.

Frequency of urination

Needing to pass water all the time can be annoying but may be the only clue that you're pregnant. The increase in urination occurs as the blood volume in your body increases, meaning you will produce more waste fluid. Also, as the womb grows to accommodate your developing foetus, it can put pressure on the neighbouring bladder, making its capacity a lot less.

The need to urinate also occurs more commonly at night as the excess fluid in your lower limbs is encouraged to drain away while you are lying in bed. Apart from causing tiredness the next day, it is a healthy sign of pregnancy.

If you are urinating even more frequently, it may be possible that you have a water infection. If you are having difficulty passing urine even though the urge is there and you are experiencing pain when passing water, you should see your doctor as you may need antibiotic medication.

Pregnancy tests

If you suspect that you may be pregnant, the best thing to do is to take a pregnancy test. If you are unsure of how to take one, don't worry – millions of women take pregnancy tests every day without knowing this information. However, it can be useful to know how your test works as it will help you understand your pregnancy and may contribute to your pregnancy experience overall.

What are they?

Pregnancy tests can be taken at home as a type of urine test or may be done by a nurse, midwife or doctor as either a urine test or blood test.

Most women in modern Britain take a test at home before they present their doctor with a positive result. Some GP surgeries will ask you to take a home test before you ask them to confirm it anyway.

Pregnancy tests can be bought from supermarkets, chemists, local convenience stores, online or even from some petrol stations. Some are expensive, others are cheaper, some contain one test, others offer you more. The choice is very wide and can be a little confusing for the user.

Spend some time reading the packets before making your purchase so that you understand exactly how each specific test works and how to use it.

Some varieties require the user to watch for a blue line appearing in one or more windows, while others give a digital display that states whether you are pregnant or not.

How do they work?

Pregnancy tests are a chemical investigation where the device is seeking the presence of a naturally made substance called human chorionic gonadotropin (hCG). This chemical is made by the developing placenta after an egg has been fertilised and implanted into the wall of the womb. Following the sixth day of fertilisation (approximately), the placenta begins to grow, supplying your foetus with all the blood, oxygen and nutrients it needs while it grows throughout pregnancy.

The amount of hCG in the body doubles around every two days following fertilisation, so the test is more accurate a week or two following fertilisation than it is within just a few days. This is why a test should ideally be taken after a period has been missed as enough time will have elapsed to give an accurate result. It also explains why the test should be repeated a week after a negative test if you are sure you might be pregnant.

'It is often the anticipation and expectation that is harder to manage than taking the test itself.'

How to take one

Pregnancy tests are very easy to take, and scientific development has made them extremely reliable and user-friendly. It is often the anticipation and expectation that is harder to manage than taking the test itself.

It can be helpful to buy a packet containing two tests as you may feel you want to repeat the test in a few days to confirm or rule out a pregnancy. Pregnancy tests can vary significantly in cost but they all have the same function and work in more or less the same way, so the cost is often quite irrelevant.

Before taking the test, make sure you are calm and ready as this will make the process easier. It may help to have a friend or family member with you when you are about to take the test, especially if you are unsure of how you will react to the result.

It is preferable to take the test first thing in the morning. This is because the hCG level tends to be higher at this time as the urine is more concentrated.

Tests normally involve the user passing a small amount of urine onto the tip of a stick which should then be left for a minute or two while the hormone registers.

Traditional tests normally show one line for a negative result and two lines for a positive result. However, you must make sure you read the packaging for each individual test's instructions and mode of mechanism.

Don't worry if you have been taking any medications as these do not affect the result unless you have been having fertility treatment and taking hormones as part of your treatment.

If you have a negative result, you probably aren't pregnant but may want to repeat the test in a few days just to make sure; it may be too early for the hormone to have registered.

If you have received a positive result, congratulations! You are pregnant and now have a lot to think about.

Telling your doctor you are pregnant

Once you have received a positive result, your emotions will be high. There will be people you'll want to tell immediately and others you won't want to tell until you have seen your doctor or had your first scan. Remember, this is your pregnancy and the decisions you make with your partner are yours alone. There is no right or wrong way to disclose your news; you will know when the time is right.

Some women panic when they get a positive result and want to rush to the doctor immediately. Although you must tell your doctor soon and book in as an antenatal patient, it isn't so urgent that you need to go and see them on the same day.

It can be helpful to phone your GP surgery, tell them you have achieved a positive pregnancy test result and ask their advice on when to book an appointment. This is because some surgeries require you to have missed two periods before you book in as this confirms the pregnancy further. The unfortunate thing about modern pregnancy tests is that they can give a positive result after just a week or two following conception, meaning that some women may not have even missed one period.

It is estimated that up to half of fertilisations do not result in a full term pregnancy and that false positive test results can and do occur, although this is rare.

'Now is the time to think about your diet, lifestyle and start reading up on pregnancy, childbirth and parenting.'

Seeing your doctor

When you attend your appointment with your doctor, it will be helpful to have a full bladder because you may be asked to do another test. However, some surgeries prefer to take a blood sample.

You will be referred to the local midwifery team who will contact you in the near future to arrange a preliminary visit, either in your own home or in a clinic.

Now is the time to think about your diet and lifestyle and start reading up on pregnancy, childbirth and parenting.

Summing Up

Discovering you are pregnant will probably trigger an entire spectrum of emotions which can range from panic to elation. Once you have confirmed your pregnancy, you may decide to tell people immediately or wait until after your first scan or check-up when you feel confident that everything is going well.

To discover your pregnancy you will need to take a test, as this is the most secure way of guaranteeing your concerns. It is likely that you will experience some of the typical symptoms before your suspicions have been confirmed.

Missing a period is the most common sign of pregnancy, however breast tenderness, nausea and vomiting, lethargy and strong desires for certain food or drink can all occur in the early months.

'Discovering you are pregnant will probably trigger an entire spectrum of emotions which can range from panic to elation.'

Once you have taken a test with a positive result, you should make an appointment with your GP. They can then refer you to a midwife who will assume responsibility for your care.

It is wise to consider taking a pregnancy test if:

■ Your period is over a week late.

■ You feel more tired than normal.

■ You need to empty your bladder more frequently.

■ You have unexplained nausea and vomiting.

■ You breasts feel more tender than normal, even before your period.

Chapter Three

The First Trimester

You have had a positive pregnancy test which has been confirmed by your doctor. Now you are wondering what exactly has happened to your body and, more importantly, what happens next.

During the first trimester there are an immense number of changes occurring in your body, most of which you are probably unaware of as they cannot be felt at this stage.

Initially, you may not even feel as though you are pregnant and can be slightly disappointed by this. Don't worry – there are several dramatic changes that do happen a little further down the road, so spend this time preparing and planning for them.

Conception and implantation

The occurrence of conception is considered by experts to be something of a miracle, as the biological processes that cause a female egg to become fertilised by a male sperm are quite amazing. This is something that most people do not spend much time thinking about, but when it is explained they are fascinated by the whole process and happy to learn that little bit more about their own body, their growing baby and how it came to exist.

Ovulation

Ovulation is something that happens every month in a normal female body, beginning in puberty and lasting until the menopause.

'During the first trimester there are an immense number of changes occurring in your body, most of which you are probably unaware of as they cannot be felt at this stage.'

Initiated by chemical releases in the ovaries, glands and the brain, the eggs (or ovum) are matured in the ovaries each month. When one is instructed to be released (again due to chemical reactions and responses), the ripest of the eggs is released by a structure called a follicle in the ovary, following which it is caught by a structure called the fimbrial end which is attached to the fallopian tube. The egg travels down the fallopian tube until it nears the internal entrance of the womb. Most eggs released remain unfertilised and are emitted from or absorbed into the body.

A healthy egg can survive for up to 24 hours in the body while waiting for a sperm to come and fertilise it, after which it dies. Sperm, however, can live for several days inside the female body, either in the vagina, the womb or the fallopian tubes. Couples who are trying to get pregnant should be having unprotected sex in the days leading up to ovulation and during the ovulatory phase itself. Waiting for an egg to be released and then having sex narrows the chances of conception; the time frame open for the sperm to find the egg before it dies is smaller.

'A healthy egg can survive for up to 24 hours in the body while waiting for a sperm to come and fertilise it.'

Fertilisation

When the sperm are released during an ejaculation, the strongest will aim for the womb and the fallopian tubes where they hope to find an egg. If the egg has been released, the strongest and most healthy sperm will try and penetrate it by 'cracking' through the outer shell, which occurs as chemicals are emitted by the sperm to make a path to the centre of the egg. Once a sperm has fertilised the egg, other sperm are unable to penetrate it. Once penetrated, the egg is known as a zygote.

When cell division begins, the outer edge of the cells form what are known as chorionic villi. They exist to attach the cells to the internal walls of the womb and also release the hormone hCG (presence of this is tested for during a pregnancy test). The zygote attaches itself firmly to the wall of the womb and can now be called a blastocyst. This whole process is called implantation.

What happens during conception?

The term conception refers to the process of fertilisation and implantation. Many women state that they can tell you exactly when they conceived, however this is probably impossible. They usually mean they can remember the sexual encounter that resulted in the pregnancy, but sperm can live in the vagina and female reproductive organs for up to 72 hours, so fertilisation could have taken place at any point during this time span.

Improving your chances of conception

There are several ways in which women and men can improve the chances of conception.

Diet and lifestyle play a large role in the successfulness of conception. Cigarette smoke is particularly harmful and has been proven to decrease the blood and oxygen supply to the reproductive organs which can affect fertility.

It can be helpful to learn how your monthly cycle works and to document the days, dates and duration of when you bleed for a few months so you can find out when you are going to ovulate.

Opinions on whether sexual position improves the chances of conception vary. In general, experts agree that the sperm should have as short a distance to travel as possible in order to have enough energy to reach the fallopian tubes. Therefore, the sperm should be ejaculated as close to the cervix as possible. It is also agreed that comfort and mental health play a role, and both partners should enjoy each other, have fun and, most importantly, be relaxed when making love.

What happens during implantation?

The process of implantation may help determine how successfully the pregnancy develops. This part of conception does not solely rely on how healthy the blastocyst is but also depends on how well the endometrium (the inner lining of the womb) has prepared itself to receive the blastocyst. Initially, it must make sure it is thick enough to accommodate the blastocyst, then get ready to secrete substances into it and provide it with a good blood supply.

The blastocyst buries itself into the wall of the womb upon which hCG is secreted and a positive pregnancy test can be gained. The blastocyst is now known as an embryo.

Lifestyle changes

Hopefully you will have been planning your pregnancy and have taken steps to ensure the best of health for both you and your growing baby. If not, all is not lost as it is never too late to make healthy changes for the benefit of you both.

Although most miscarriages do happen during these tentative weeks, making positive changes can significantly improve the chances of your pregnancy progressing.

'Your diet is extremely important during the entire pregnancy and in the best circumstances should be taken into account before conception occurs.'

Changing your diet

Your diet is extremely important during the entire pregnancy and in the best circumstances should be taken into account before conception occurs. However, it is never too late to start taking more care with your diet, whether you are pregnant or not.

During the first trimester it is very important to make sure you are still taking enough folic acid in your diet. As mentioned in chapter 1, this mineral is vital in the early development of your baby and without it many very serious and long term problems can occur. Taking a supplement is the easiest and best way of ensuring you are getting enough.

Feeling sick

Feeling sick during the first few months is very common. Unfortunately, there is often little you can do about it other than to simply ride it out and wait until it eases. The good news is that it normally stops or decreases in severity after the first trimester, when you will start to feel really healthy again.

Don't worry about this sickness – many women who endure it worry whether it is going to have a negative effect on their baby but go on to have extremely healthy pregnancies and children.

Avoid foods that make you queasy; sometimes even the smell or the thought of a certain food can make you feel nauseous, so don't force yourself to make something (even if it is your or your partner's favourite!).

Try snacking on ginger biscuits – ginger products are well known for their benefits of lessening the feeling of nausea.

If, however, you cannot even keep fluids down, you must tell your doctor or midwife as there is a risk of becoming dehydrated which is no good for the health of you or your baby. In extreme cases, you may have to have fluids through a drip for a few days and some anti-sickness medications until you are feeling better.

Cutting down on alcohol

The subject of alcohol and pregnancy has been discussed at length in recent years. Initially, experts suggested that no alcohol should be consumed during a pregnancy. This was then followed by advice that staying within the recommended amounts of one unit once or twice a week will do no harm. However, it should be noted that alcohol is absorbed directly into the bloodstream, after which it is transferred through the placenta to your baby, so your baby has to drink whatever you drink. Babies cannot process alcohol like adults, and the damage of exceeding these limits is very well known. It can range from developmental defects to causing miscarriage or premature births.

According to the Department of Health 'pregnant women or women trying to conceive should avoid drinking alcohol. If you do choose to drink, to protect the baby, you should not drink more than one to two units of alcohol once or twice a week and you should not get drunk.' For more information, visit www. dh.gov.uk.

Pelvic floor exercises

The pelvic floor is the name given to the network of muscles that help keep your pelvic organs in the right place. These muscles and ligaments can become damaged by many things, including weight gain and excessive strain.

It is no secret that your pelvic floor is probably going to be affected by either the pregnancy or the birth itself (probably both), so you really should take steps to protect it and prevent any long term damage before your pelvis changes too much.

Among other things, a damaged pelvic floor can cause problems with bladder continence, so please try and take some preventative measures.

Ask your midwife or practice nurse how to do pelvic floor exercises. They are easy and can be done anywhere without anyone knowing you are doing them.

Dealing with tiredness

'Ask your midwife or practice nurse how to do pelvic floor exercises. They are easy and can be done anywhere without anyone knowing you are doing them.'

Some women feel perfectly healthy all the way through pregnancy, while some suffer with symptoms and pregnancy associated complaints for the whole nine months. Some women find that they only suffer from the symptoms during the first trimester – this is very common.

Most women will admit that they felt more tired, even exhausted, during the first 12 weeks than at any other time during the pregnancy. Your body is experiencing huge changes during this time, and the activity that is going on in your body has to be supplied with energy from the mother while the embryo establishes itself and grows into a foetus.

The tiredness can be quite a surprise for some women, who feel disappointed that they are not 'blossoming' in their pregnancy as they thought they would.

You may find that you need to sleep a lot more than normal, have no energy to do the things you did before you were pregnant and wonder how you will cope when the baby comes. Don't worry, this tiredness is temporary and a normal part of the first trimester.

It is important to allow your body to dictate how you respond to the tiredness. If you don't feel like going out, don't. Give yourself the luxury of resting when you can. Make sure you take your break entitlements at work, and put your feet up with a drink and a snack to re-charge your batteries.

When to tell people you are pregnant

There are no right or wrong ways to tell others you are pregnant. While some women are comfortable telling everyone their news as soon as they find out, others like to wait until they have fully absorbed the discovery themselves.

Traditionally, women liked to wait until they had confirmation from their healthcare provider or had attended their first scan or appointment, but in recent times more and more women and couples are sharing their news as soon as they find out.

It's your choice

When you first see the positive result of a pregnancy test, you will probably feel a little overwhelmed, elated or even quite anxious. Sharing this news is a huge occurrence for some people, and the circumstance of the pregnancy will affect how they feel about telling others.

It is your pregnancy and your choice as to who you tell first. You don't need to decide immediately who you are going to tell first and who you are going to wait to tell.

'It is your pregnancy and your choice as to who you tell first.'

Sometimes it can be beneficial to wait to tell other people until you have had time to digest the feeling of being pregnant and exactly how you feel about it. Some women like to plan how they are going to disclose the news, many preferring to do it face to face or in a group rather than over the phone or simply letting it travel through conversation and gossip.

You are not obliged to follow any particular pattern of behaviour and can tell whoever you like, whenever you like.

Telling your partner

Telling your partner or the father of the child that you are expecting can feel particularly daunting for some women as they are unsure of what sort of reaction to expect. This is especially true if the pregnancy has not been planned or they are not in a relationship with that person any more. If you are in a similar situation, it may be better to wait until you are 100% sure of your pregnancy and know exactly what your plans are.

If you are in a very stable relationship, you may tell your partner that you suspect you are pregnant as soon as you miss a period. This may mean they await the result of the pregnancy test with you and you share the news as a couple, or that they come with you when you attend your first appointment. This can be very beneficial as it helps the father connect with their future baby at a very early stage, and it may be a memory that they treasure throughout their whole life.

Before or after the first scan?

It is common for a lot of couples to keep their news to themselves until they have had their first scan, as this is normally performed at the end of the first trimester when the pregnancy is over the most risky stage. Also, a scan can provide reassurance to the couple that their baby is developing as expected and can predict a date for when the baby is due.

Modern pregnancy tests, however, can be taken extremely early on in the pregnancy, and many couples find that they simply can't wait until the scan to tell everyone of the pregnancy. There is nothing wrong with telling people straightaway. One issue that should be taken into account, however, is that many pregnancies discovered very early on may not progress to a first stage scan, meaning that the good news and elation may be short lived.

Telling your employer you are pregnant

When you first find out you are pregnant, you may feel it is safer to tell your employer straightaway. This is especially true if you work in an area that may pose a risk to either the health of you or your baby. In occupations such as those which include a lot of manual handling, work with chemicals or x-rays or other high risk areas, you may feel that it is best to disclose the information to your organisation early on. Your employer should treat this information as confidential and risk-assess your workplace for safety during pregnancy. When required, alternative duties should be encouraged and this should not affect your rights as an employee.

Your growing foetus

The changes going on in your lower abdomen during the first trimester are immense. Unfortunately, because you don't change shape very much or feel any different, you are unaware of what is going on. Rest assured that there is plenty of activity happening, involving both the growing foetus and your body.

The amniotic sac

The amniotic sac is formed during the first trimester. This is the protective membrane that encases the baby for the whole pregnancy. It is actually made up of two membranes called the amnion and the chorion, and contains amniotic fluid. The baby moves around in the amniotic fluid, as well as being cushioned by it and protected from any injuries.

The placenta

The placenta is made very early on in the pregnancy and connects the baby to the mother's womb via the umbilical cord. Within the placenta all forms of nutrients are exchanged from the mother to the baby, and waste products made by the baby are transferred back to the mother's bloodstream. It is a very important organ in the pregnancy and any problems with it can risk both the mother and the baby.

The umbilical cord

The umbilical cord is a rope-like structure that directly connects the baby to the placenta and is comprised of blood vessels that are responsible for the exchange of oxygen, nutrients and waste. It is quite long in length and can pose a risk to the baby during the late stages of pregnancy and labour as it can easily wrap around the baby's neck.

First trimester benchmarks

During the first trimester there are many benchmarks that your baby will reach that are essential to its development.

For example, in the first four weeks the first stages of the brain and spinal cord develop, the beginnings of the circulatory and digestive systems form and even the limbs start to grow.

After eight weeks, your embryo can now be called a foetus. It has started to take a more human shape and has even started to develop tooth buds. The nose and mouth have started to take form, and your foetus is quite happy moving around in its sac (even though it cannot be felt). By now it may be as big as one and a half inches in size.

'During the first trimester there are many benchmarks that your baby will reach that are essential to its development.'

Antenatal check-ups

When you have had your pregnancy confirmed and have informed your GP or GP practice that you are pregnant, you will be advised to undergo some tests and check-ups in the antenatal stages, particularly if this is your first pregnancy. These tests and appointments exist for three main reasons. Firstly, your overall health and understanding of pregnancy will be assessed. This is to make sure you know what to expect in the coming months, and to make sure you have no problems that may be detrimental to the pregnancy. Secondly, the health of your developing baby will be monitored so that any problems can be detected and acted upon as early as possible, giving both you and your baby the best possible health for the future. Lastly, they exist to prepare you for the pregnancy and the birth of your baby, and to explain all the options and choices you have with regard to your condition.

Your first appointment

Your first appointment is extremely important as it not only books you into the antenatal care pathway that is implemented in your region, but allows your midwife to assess the likelihood of any problems that may occur. It also offers you the chance to ask any questions you may have.

You will be asked to provide a detailed personal medical history and disclose any illnesses that have been found in either your parents or your partner's parents. Sometimes it may not be possible to find out this information so don't worry too much, but the more information you can provide, the better your midwife can plan care for both you and your baby.

You will also need to tell your midwife of any past pregnancies, stillbirths or miscarriages, along with any gynaecological problems you have had.

Blood screening tests

Your blood will be tested for many reasons, the most important one being to determine your blood group.

All women are now tested for their 'rhesus factor', in other words – to find out whether you are a positive or negative blood group. If you are positive and your partner is negative, you may have a baby who is also negative, in which case your blood and the baby's blood types are incompatible and you may naturally produce antibodies against the baby. This can be successfully treated as long as your rhesus compatibility has been established and provisions made for it.

Other reasons for having blood taken are to screen for any genetic problems, any existing infections (including sexually transmitted infections) and to determine if there are any existing illnesses or any history of conditions such as rubella.

Weight, height and urine checks

Your weight and urine will probably be checked at each appointment you attend during the whole pregnancy. These measurements are taken to find out if you are gaining weight, whether you have a healthy weight for your frame and to detect any blood, glucose, protein or other substances in your urine. These substances could be a sign of an underlying problem like a urine infection, which can be dangerous during pregnancy.

'When you have had your pregnancy confirmed and have informed your GP or GP practice that you are pregnant, you will be advised to undergo some tests and check-ups in the antenatal stages, particularly if this is your first pregnancy.'

Palpation and listening to the baby's heart rate

Most women are very excited but also slightly nervous during the first few appointments as they want to be reassured that everything is okay, and most ask if they are able to listen to the baby's heart rate using the equipment used by the midwife.

In most cases, it isn't a problem to hear the baby's heart rate (as long as the equipment is available), and usually this is enough to give women the assurance they need that their baby is developing normally.

Don't panic if you hear a very fast heart rate as this is perfectly healthy for your baby. Ideally, it should be around 100, plus the mother's heart rate, per minute.

Your midwife will also want to examine your abdomen and feel the top of your womb. Although this can be uncomfortable, it is necessary and will be used as a growth measurement during your next appointment.

Summing Up

A pregnancy is divided into three parts: the first trimester, the second trimester and the third trimester.

The first trimester refers to the time between your last period and the end of the twelfth week. During this time your body is going through enormous changes and your baby is well on his or her way to being almost fully formed, though very small.

Both you and your baby are working hard to ensure that his or her environment and internal organs are developing correctly and are in working order. Your baby has begun to sprout limbs and even has the beginning of dentistry.

You will probably undergo many tests including blood tests, blood pressure checks, weight and height assessments, urine tests and a scan. These tests are all necessary to pick up any early warning signs and to make sure the correct treatment plan can be scheduled for the benefit of both you and your baby.

'Both you and your baby are working hard to ensure that his or her environment and internal organs are developing correctly and are in working order.'

Chapter Four

The Second Trimester

Congratulations! You are now in your second trimester and can start to relax, enjoy your pregnancy and make plans for the arrival of your baby.

Most women usually find that some of the more uncomfortable or unpleasant aspects at the beginning of the pregnancy are starting to subside, and they are generally feeling healthier and finding the experience more pleasurable.

The second trimester is full of changes and developments for both mother and baby. During this time your body adapts and changes size and shape and you will start to 'look' pregnant as your tummy grows. You will also be able to relate to your baby when you first start to feel it move; a very special and unique occurrence for all pregnant women.

You will often be requested to attend appointments every four to six weeks until you get closer to your due date. However, this general rule may vary if you have any conditions that require closer assessment or you are having any problems.

Your changing body

Now is the time you can really start enjoying your pregnancy as you are over the danger zone and are starting to show the beginnings of a new life. People are very receptive to the good news of pregnancy, so enjoy it while you can and allow yourself to start getting excited and planning for your little one.

'During this time your body adapts and changes size and shape and you will start to "look" pregnant as your tummy grows.'

Stretch marks

Many women worry desperately about getting stretch marks, how bad they will be and whether they will disappear after the baby is born. Unfortunately, this is one of the unpleasant parts of pregnancy and affects almost all pregnant women at some point.

There are several old wives tales about preventing or reducing stretch marks, but so far medical research has proven to be of little use regarding their prevention. The simple answer is that even though you can smother your skin from head to toe with the most expensive moisturisers in the world, this may act as no defence against the marks. It really depends on your type of skin and your genetics. Many midwives agree that the chances of getting stretch marks increase if your own mother had them, though this is still no concrete guarantee.

'It is useful to make sure you have a few comfortable bras in your drawer that you know will give you support and will allow for your breasts to grow.'

They can occur during any stage of the pregnancy and tend to worsen as your body grows with your bump. You may find them on your abdomen, your breasts, your hips and thighs and even on your back and arms. They begin as red or purple lines that vary in thickness and depth, and happen as your skin stretches and cannot cope with the excessive tension. These lines will fade over time and become less noticeable but can still usually be seen if examined closely.

The only products that have proven to help lessen their severity are those containing vitamin E derivatives and those that have been specifically designed to reduce the appearance of scars and other skin blemishes.

Your breasts

Your breasts are a very important part of the pregnancy and can change in just a few weeks. They will often change in size, weight and appearance and will become sensitive, sometimes painful, and start producing milk even before the birth. Most women like having more rounded, larger breasts, so don't be afraid to enjoy them!

It is useful to make sure you have a few comfortable bras in your drawer that you know will give you support but will still allow for your breasts to grow. It is also likely that you will need to buy a few new bras as your pregnancy develops. If you are planning to breastfeed, it may be cost-effective to buy nursing bras that assist with breastfeeding, even before you need to use them in this way.

Your nipples will usually become more prominent (expect this to increase when breastfeeding) and the area around the nipple will darken. This often fades quite a lot after breastfeeding has ceased but may still leave the area slightly darker than before the pregnancy.

If your breasts were extremely painful during the first part of your pregnancy, it is likely that the pain will lessen during the second trimester (although if it continues, it's still a healthy sign). Many women find that the increased sensitivity adds to their romantic life, while others find the pain too much to bear. If you find it uncomfortable, tell your partner to spend more time touching other areas.

Many women find that their veins become more prominent and a brighter shade of blue during the pregnancy, especially during the second trimester. This occurs because the blood supply to the breast tissue increases as the demand for blood, nutrients and oxygen is higher.

As your milk supply begins to develop, you may find that you start to lose a milky substance from your nipples. This is called colostrum and is the first stage of milk that your newborn needs to thrive. Don't worry about leaking it now – you will continue to produce it until your baby doesn't need it anymore or until you start to use formula feeds. Many supermarkets and chemists now sell affordable absorbent breast pads that can be placed in the bra to stop the fluid leaking onto your clothes and becoming noticeable.

Pelvic pain

If all the other changes in your body weren't enough, you may also experience some degree of pelvic pain – no one said pregnancy was a walk in the park!

Towards the latter half of the second trimester and entering the third, as your pelvis struggles to cope with a rapidly growing womb, you may find some discomfort as your other lower organs need to find a new position for the next few months. This can take some shuffling about and can make you feel a little nauseous and bloated. Don't worry – it will settle. However, just as it does, along comes another source of discomfort! The ligaments that hold everything in place start to soften and loosen in preparation for the work that needs to be done when the womb gets even larger. It is helpful to have a really positive mental attitude during these times and embrace the changes as part of a healthy pregnancy and try to take it all in your stride. If, however, you are feeling very uncomfortable, please tell your midwife who may be able to suggest some exercises that will help alleviate the discomfort.

In general, it is useful to take exercise at this stage as it will help lessen any back pain (which is common), ease the labour and decrease the after effects of the pregnancy. Yoga, pilates and swimming can be particularly good forms of exercise for pregnant women.

'Your baby is now well on the way to developing the features that it will be born with and much of the intricate physical development is complete.'

If, however, at any time during the pregnancy you feel any sharp pains in your pelvis, pains that do not ease after a few hours or any pain that is accompanied by bleeding, seek medical attention urgently, even if it only serves to ease your mind.

Your growing baby

Your baby is now well on the way to developing the features that it will be born with and much of the intricate physical development is complete. Sometimes you will actually be able to make out his or her facial features and characteristics on the scans you have during the pregnancy.

The amniotic sac, placenta and umbilical cord

The fluid in the sac continues to increase and will protect and surround the baby until the membranes are ruptured during labour. It does, however, change slightly as the baby uses the fluid to practise necessary functions, such as lung movements, and produces tiny amounts of urine (which means the baby's kidneys are beginning to work).

The placenta continues to provide vital life to your baby and is increasing in size. In fact, it is measured along with your baby during the scans to help determine the size and approximate gestation of the pregnancy.

During the scans your placenta will be assessed to make sure it is not in a dangerous position, such as lying low in the womb or over the cervix. It is also assessed to make sure it is still fully adhered to the inside of your womb and has not come away in any place. This could severely compromise the health of your baby as it means there is the potential for decreased oxygen and nutrients reaching the placenta.

Second trimester benchmarks

The second trimester is an exciting time for foetal development. At around 14 weeks your baby is moving around in its sac with some vigour, though it is unlikely you will feel these just yet (subsequent pregnancies may allow you to feel these movements earlier than the first). Your baby will even be able to change its facial expression and may experience some episodes of hiccups.

At around 16 weeks the baby's eyebrows and hair start to grow, and the eyes start responding to light outside the womb. This means your baby may start to distinguish night from day. This is shortly followed by the sense of hearing developing, so your baby will now be able to hear your voice and sometimes those of people around you.

By week 20, babies can weigh around half a pound in weight and their fat layers are starting to accumulate.

Towards the end of this trimester, your baby will start to use their lungs and will prepare for breathing air by practising inhaling and exhaling the fluid in the amniotic sac. It is also likely that he or she will have defined footprints and fingerprints, making them totally unique.

Week 24 is very important as it is at this time that your baby may stand a chance of survival if they are born early, though this cannot be guaranteed.

'As your tummy expands and begins to become more noticeable, you may find that you have to make certain changes and allowances to maintain your safety and comfort.'

Adapting to your bump

As your tummy expands and begins to become more noticeable, you may find that you have to make certain changes and allowances to maintain your safety and comfort.

Certain daily tasks like fastening your shoes, putting your seat belt on in the car or reaching to the top shelf in the kitchen cupboard may become more difficult. Even silly things like doing the ironing and getting in and out of the bath will not come as easily as they once did.

Your safety is paramount, so standing on chairs or worktops to reach things is certainly not a good idea. Instead, try and adapt your environment if you can. Remember, your bump is going to continue growing and will eventually prevent you from doing some of the things you once took for granted, so you'll need to find new ways of doing things for a while.

Maternity clothes and where to get them

In the past, maternity clothes were notoriously frumpy and quite difficult to get hold of. Nowadays, fortunately, things have changed. High street shops and supermarkets (the ones that stock clothes) are now very good at designing fashionable but comfortable clothing ranges with the expectant mother in mind. Their profile is further endorsed by the use of models and celebrities advertising the clothes which can be brought at affordable prices.

There are also many more exclusive, hence more expensive, boutiques and shops that are aimed solely at the pregnant woman and can offer designer labels. But unless you can easily afford them, there are probably other more sensible ways of spending your money – remember, babies can be costly!

If you are on a very tight budget, try looking on the Internet for ideas. There are many websites that offer an exchange or sales service where women can sell their unwanted maternity clothes for a fraction of the price that the shops may offer. As the clothes are only worn for a few months, they are generally in good condition and are probably still quite fashionable.

Sleeping comfortably

Even though you may have previously been the world's greatest sleeper, pregnancy can change your habits and ability to get comfy. Likewise, you may feel more comfortable and secure with a bump than before because you are more content with your life and are looking forward to having an addition to your family.

If you are having difficulty finding a comfortable sleeping position, here are some tips that may help.

- It is advisable that you start sleeping on your left side if you are able to as this keeps the circulation of both you and your baby healthy. Lying on your right may encourage some of the major blood vessels to become compressed. It is, however, important to not let this become too much of an issue during the early part of the second trimester (or keep you awake worrying about it). Getting into the habit now merely helps you get used to it for when it does become more important later on.

- Often the easiest way to get to sleep is to make sure you are comfortable by wearing nightwear that is suitable. Tight fitting or non-supportive clothes may hinder you; nightdresses and loose drawstring or elasticated pyjamas can do wonders for your comfort.

- If you have an understanding and accommodating partner, perhaps a massage may not be out of the question, especially if you are looking for intimacy without wanting intercourse.

Sleeping should be slightly easier at this stage as you are less likely to have a lot of caffeine in your body and now need to take fewer toilet breaks during the night.

Feeling protective of your bump

You may not know it but your maternal instinct has probably already kicked in. There are several occasions when women worry about and think primarily of their bump, often putting it before their own needs. This is perfectly natural and is the beginning of that very special bond you will have with your baby.

There are, however, certain circumstances in which women may find they get frustrated, and again this is natural. The general public seem to have a need to give pregnant women special attention, which is nice, and rightly so in most circumstances, but it can be irritating. People may try and touch your bump when they greet you; this may be a natural reaction for them but can be highly annoying for you! If you really don't like strangers touching you or feel threatened, try and avoid the situation.

'It is advisable that you start sleeping on your left side if you are able to as this keeps the circulation of both you and your baby healthy.'

When you approach people, have your own hands on your bump thus showing people there is no room for them to touch. Perhaps you could try and stand to the side so that your bump is not so inviting and you are not as exposed as you would be if you were facing forward. If you really aren't getting anywhere and still hate the idea, politely tell people that you don't like it and would they mind not touching you. Let's face it, in what other circumstances would we let a stranger touch us?

Check-ups and appointments

'Your check-ups and appointments are extremely important, and while many women and their partners look forward to finding out that everything is going well, it is natural to feel slightly nervous.'

Your check-ups and appointments are extremely important, and while many women and their partners look forward to finding out that everything is going well, it is natural to feel slightly nervous.

Always remember to jot down any questions you may want to ask your midwife or doctor when they occur to you – by the time the appointment has come, you are likely to have forgotten; pregnancy plays havoc with your memory!

When you go for your appointments, try and have a drink before you go as you will probably be asked to provide a urine sample when you get there.

Remember to take your medical and/or midwifery notes with you as your midwife will need to document your latest test results and compare them to your previous ones to detect any changes.

Feeling your baby move

Feeling your baby move is very special. Only you will know what this feels like, and although women have been having babies for thousands of years, feeling your own baby move and learning its patterns is something that no one else will experience. It is a very good way of starting to bond with your baby.

It is important to feel your baby move as this is a sign of healthy foetal development and will reassure you that everything is fine.

Was it a kick or not?

It is around the 18 week mark (sometimes slightly earlier or later than this) that you will first feel your baby move. The first movements may not be very noticeable and may be mistaken for wind, muscular twitches or normal bowel movements as they are not normally distinguishable kicks. Many women compare the feelings to a flutter and like a butterfly in their tummy, sometimes like a tickle.

You may have noticed on your first scan that your baby is extremely active and wonder why you can't feel it. Soon you will be able to, and it's not quite how people imagine. Your tiny baby is twisting, turning and enjoying being able to wriggle in your womb, and all you may feel at first is a minor quiver that doesn't feel a true representation of all the activity going on inside.

As the weeks pass, the movements become stronger and more apparent and will continue right up until the birth. In the later weeks you will be able to see definite movements simply by looking at your tummy.

Your partner may also enjoy feeling the baby move and will be able to do so by placing a hand on your tummy and being patient until the baby decides to say hello.

Understanding your baby's body clock

Believe it or not, but you may be able to determine your baby's body clock while it is still developing inside you. More often than not, you will feel your baby awake at night having a good wriggle around but being quiet and content during the day. This may be so, yet it is more likely that the movements are there during the day but you are too busy to feel them or are getting used to feeling them. When you are in bed at night or in the bath, you are more relaxed and therefore more likely to feel them.

Many women worry that their baby is awake at night and think that they will have a baby who won't sleep when it is born. Don't worry – there is no evidence to suggest that babies who seem to be more active at night follow the same pattern after they are born.

'It is important to feel your baby move as this is a sign of healthy foetal development and will reassure you that everything is fine.'

Counting the movements

When your foetal movements are established and you are used to the movement and any noticeable patterns, it is possible to keep a diary of them. This is called kick count monitoring.

From around seven months onwards, it is a good idea to start learning the patterns and what is normal for your baby. By doing this you will be able to detect early on if your baby's movements have decreased or stopped altogether. Although this is rare, it may be a sign that you need assessing by your midwife and a quick check-up will put your mind at ease.

Keep a small notepad to hand in which you can document your baby's movements. Although you will probably never need to refer to this (unless either you or your midwife are worried), it can make a very good keepsake of your pregnancy.

However, it should be remembered that busy working women may not always be able to keep track of the movements and may not notice them so much when they are busy. If you are active, you may not notice the movements as they are hard to distinguish from your own. Try not to worry too much if you haven't noticed any movements for a few hours as they can be monitored at a more appropriate time, and in most cases they have been happening but have not been detected.

Need2Know

Summing Up

The second trimester is determined as weeks 13 to 28 and by now you will really start to look and feel pregnant.

Your baby is now growing quite rapidly and this alters the shape of your body. You may find that your skin is getting quite stretched and starting to develop stretch marks, and your breasts are getting larger and starting to feel full.

By the middle of the second trimester you should start to feel your baby moving around in the womb, even though he or she has been very active since much earlier on.

Initially, this may be mistaken for something else, but by the end of the second trimester you will know exactly when your baby is having a wriggle and will probably be quite comforted by the experience.

It is at this stage that you may have to start adapting your life around your bump as sleeping, standing and your exercise regime may need to be amended.

All of the uncomfortable symptoms that you experienced in the first trimester are now gone and you can really start to enjoy the pregnancy. Your hair is probably getting thicker and glossier and your nails may be in a much better condition (although this is not the case for everyone).

'It is at this stage that you may have to start adapting your life around your bump as sleeping, standing and your exercise regime may need to be amended.'

Chapter Five

The Third Trimester

Well done! You have reached the final trimester of your pregnancy and you can really begin to prepare for your new arrival.

You are probably now looking like a pregnant woman and are spending much of your time discussing baby-related subjects or talking about pregnancy and birth with your friends.

The third trimester is the time between the seventh and ninth month of the pregnancy and many women now feel that the end of this particular journey is in sight.

Your body

Your body will continue to undergo exciting changes, although at this stage it is more in preparation for the birth. Your baby is now already developed and will use these last few weeks mainly to increase in size and weight to ensure they have the healthiest start after birth.

For many women, the pregnancy only becomes obvious in this last phase. Their bump becomes more prominent and they start to feel some of the changes that occur as both their body and the baby get ready for labour and birth.

'The third trimester is the time between the seventh and ninth month of the pregnancy and many women now feel that the end of this particular journey is in sight.'

Your breasts

It is likely that your breasts will have grown considerably during the last few weeks as they continue to produce milk supplies, and you may also find that some of this leaks. If your nipples are becoming sore, try massaging a small amount of the leakage into the nipple itself as this can help keep it moisturised and hydrated, and continue to use breast pads if needed.

You may also have noticed that the veins in your breasts are even more noticeable and worry that they may stay this way. Don't panic, as in almost all cases they return to their normal state when breast milk has ceased production.

Not all women find that their breasts change during pregnancy and worry that this means they will have difficulty with breastfeeding. However, this does not necessarily mean that you won't start making milk during labour or shortly after your baby has been delivered. Likewise, if you have inverted or flat nipples, this is not a sign that you will not be able to breastfeed. It may just mean that you will need some additional help with the first few attempts.

'The overall shape of your bump may change frequently as your baby moves around and starts to make its way into the lower part of the pelvis.'

Your bump

Your baby is now growing at quite a substantial rate and this is reflected in your swollen tummy. The overall shape of your bump may change frequently as your baby moves around and starts to make its way into the lower part of the pelvis. The movements can often be seen in the abdomen, and it may even be possible to determine what part of the baby you are looking at, for example a hand or a foot can sometimes be depicted.

Your pelvis

As your baby begins to enter the lower half of the pelvis, you may find that you are feeling a lot of pressure and aching in the lower part of your abdomen. This is not only a result of the baby's weight, but happens because the ligaments and muscles are starting to prepare for labour and often some of the major blood vessels in the area become compressed and engorged with blood.

For many, these symptoms can be eased by changing your position or taking a warm bath, while for others it is merely part of the pregnancy and must be endured until the aches have subsided in their own time.

The vulva (vaginal area) is also susceptible to some changes and you may find that your labia (vaginal lips) become enlarged and discoloured. This is normal and is simply a sign that there is a good blood supply to the area and they are getting ready for the passage of your baby.

Backache

Lower backache in the last trimester is very common and largely occurs as a result of carrying extra body weight. It can also be because the baby is lying in an awkward position and is pressing on nerves, muscles or parts of your blood supply. In this instance, the symptoms may be intermittent and subside when the baby next moves.

Backache can be eased by wearing more supportive clothing and by taking additional rest periods during the day. It may also be helpful to place a pillow behind your lower back when you are sitting or lying down.

Some light massage or a warm bath can also help ease symptoms, as can frequently changing your position. Using a small stool to place under one foot if you have to stand for long periods at work, for example, eases the pressure; alternate the stool to the other side if needed.

If you are experiencing a lot of pain, please speak to your midwife, doctor or chemist before taking any medication.

'If you are experiencing a lot of pain, please speak to your midwife, doctor or chemist before taking any medication.'

Other changes

As your baby grows, there are several other changes that might happen and are equally important to be aware of. Increased urination is common as your bladder doesn't have the same amount of room as before and can hold a lot less before it needs emptying. There is, however, also an increased risk of developing a urinary tract infection which can be dangerous if left undiagnosed and hence untreated. If your urine looks cloudy, is blood stained, smells offensive or it is taking longer to instigate urinating, please see your midwife who can perform a simple urine test to check for the presence of infection. It can be helpful to drink a glass of fresh cranberry juice every day to help prevent an infection from developing in the first instance.

It is not uncommon to find that you experience some amount of vaginal discharge towards the end of your pregnancy as the mucus in and around the cervix becomes more likely to come away. This is normal and can be controlled using panty liners. If the discharge becomes blood stained or becomes a constant trickle, please tell your midwife as this may be a sign that your membranes have started to rupture.

Retaining fluids is also part of late pregnancy and it often accumulates around the ankles and feet. This happens as the blood vessels find it harder to return the blood to your heart. It is not normally a problem and can be treated by elevating the lower limbs when possible and by wearing shoes that can be adjusted to accommodate the change in size, such as trainers. If the swelling becomes severe and you are feeling flushed and breathless, have a severe headache or are experiencing visual disturbances, please speak to your midwife urgently as your blood pressure may be creeping up which can be dangerous and will need treating.

You and your baby – third trimester benchmarks

Your baby will now have almost finished developing and will spend the remainder of the pregnancy growing in size and preparing for the outside world.

During these weeks you may find that you really start to bond with your baby and that the whole experience has become more real.

You

As your pregnancy progresses, you will start to feel tired more easily. This is because you are carrying excess weight and have such a lot of activity going on inside. Take rest when you need it.

'As your pregnancy progresses, you will start to feel tired more easily. This is because you are carrying excess weight and have such a lot of activity going on inside. Take rest when you need it.'

It is also very common to feel more sluggish and full more quickly. This can usually be remedied by taking smaller, more frequent meals, and by making sure you take time out after eating to digest properly.

If heartburn is becoming a problem, try sucking mints. It may be possible to take an over-the-counter remedy, but please make sure your chemist has advised that the preparation is safe for pregnant women.

As your baby is moving around inside, you may find it more difficult to change position and can actually feel a hand or foot sticking in your ribs. This can be alleviated by gently massaging the area to try and manipulate the baby's movement away.

By the 31 week mark, the top of your bump should be around four inches above your navel, which can cause your other internal organs to become pushed up and more uncomfortable, leaving you breathless more easily. Taking exercise is essential but you may now need to take it more slowly and warm-up and warm-down more thoroughly. Yoga, pilates and swimming are still very achievable and should be encouraged, though your instructor may have to tailor your schedule to suit your pregnancy.

As you reach the final few weeks of the pregnancy (around week 36), you may all of a sudden find that you can eat larger meals again and that your breathlessness is easing. This is because your baby is now getting ready for birth and has sunk low into your pelvis. Do not worry too much if this hasn't happened – your midwife will be checking the baby's position at each visit and will assess how far into your pelvis he or she is. If your baby is still in a head up position, you will be taught how to encourage it into a head down position, which makes for the easiest and safest birth.

Your baby

By week 30 your baby will weigh around three pounds and will be able to open and close its eyes, suck its thumb and will have fully formed fingernails. He or she will be quite happily growing in size, constantly producing millions of new nerves cells that it will need to survive.

Not only will the baby be responsive to light, it will be able to respond to sound and may even be startled by a loud or sudden noise. He or she will be developing their own little character and finding out how to do new things every day; some of these characteristics may be part of their personality once they are born.

If you are having a boy, his testis should descend into his scrotum by week 32-33, although occasionally they do not descend until after the birth or in the first year or two of life.

Within a few more weeks, your little one's immune system gets a boost as he or she begins to produce antibodies that will help fight infections once they are born.

'Talking to your baby is a great way of spending time together and establishing a good relationship, and this can begin during your pregnancy.'

The baby is around 17-18 inches in length and will gain around one pound every week from now until birth. They are nearly ready to face the world, and labour may begin at any time.

Getting ready for the birth

For the past six months to a year, you have planned, conceived and grown your baby. Now it is all about to come to the climax of the birth and meeting your little one, and it is totally natural to wonder how you will cope. A lot of your concerns can be resolved by being prepared for the event, making sure all your questions are answered and most of your fears are eased. This can be achieved by trying to plan for the event, reading up on the subject, talking to your healthcare providers, discussing things with others and attending classes that are designed for pregnant women and their partners.

Getting to know your baby before the birth

There are many ways in which you can start getting to know your baby before he or she has made their grand entrance. You may already be aware of their sleep/wake cycle (often this is the total opposite of yours!) and are taking steps to ensure the bond between you has begun.

Talking to your bump can be a very good start to the bonding process. When your baby is born and the initial few weeks have passed, you will probably find you are spending periods of time alone with them and wondering what to do. Talking to your baby is a great way of spending time together and establishing a good relationship, and this can begin during your pregnancy. The baby will already have developed a sense of hearing and will know your voice and may even respond to it already. Imagine the benefits of this when he or she is crying and can be soothed by your voice.

It is very common for women to stroke their bump as it grows, and this again is the beginning of your bond and shows your maternal and protective side. It is a great way of easing your aches and it feels as though you are comforting your baby too.

Keeping a diary is another way of bonding and sharing the experience with your child. You can keep an accurate record of your emotions and experiences that can be shared in the future, providing your child with some insight of how excited or nervous you were when they were due. Why not add some pregnancy photos too?

Making plans for the birth

Your midwife may have already discussed with you the idea of writing a birth plan. This document is a way of communicating your ideas and expectations with your healthcare providers, helping to ensure that your wishes are followed. They can include the type of birth you would like, the types of pain relief you would be happy to consider, who you want to accompany you in the delivery room, how you plan to feed your baby after the birth and any other wishes or ideas that you have.

Although it may not always be possible to follow these plans exactly, they can help you think about the birth and learn more about it, even opening up possibilities that you have previously not considered.

It is very helpful to try and be quite open about what you definitely don't want rather than being too specific about what you do want. The last thing you want is to compromise your health or that of your baby's by being too restrictive with your instructions and wishes.

If you are unsure about planning the birth, it can be useful to attend antenatal classes and learn how others are planning theirs.

You will also need to make preparations for sterilising equipment if you are planning to bottle feed your baby. The last thing you will want to do is get home from the hospital with your new baby and find that you have no provisions for feeding him or her.

You will also need to think about shopping for your new baby and buying items such as a cot, Moses' basket, pushchair or pram, bedding, clothes and nappies. It is advisable to buy only one or two packs of nappies until you have had your baby, as you don't want to have too many that are not the right size.

'It is advisable to buy only one or two packs of nappies until you have had your baby, as you don't want to have too many that are not the right size.'

Part of your birth plan should also include how you are going to get to the hospital if you are going to one, or how to contact your midwife if you are having a home birth. It is always best to make a trial visit to the hospital so that you know the best route, where to go when you get there and where the drop-off points and car parks are.

Attending classes

Antenatal classes are sessions designed specifically for the needs of expectant parents. They aim to educate people about pregnancy and the birthing process and allow for questions, discussions and experimenting with equipment. You will also be taught how to spot the first signs of labour, what to do when it begins, relaxation techniques and when you need to contact your healthcare provider. This information is also extremely useful for your partner and can provide an excellent way of allowing them to be part of the pregnancy.

Classes are usually free and available to all pregnant women and their families. As each area may offer a slightly different service to another, it is important that you ask your midwife what is available in your area and whether it is suitable for you to attend.

Packing your bag

Knowing what to pack in your hospital bag can be a tricky subject and it can be very tempting to over pack so that you are prepared for every eventuality. However, it's a lot easier than most people think. If you are having a home birth, you may still want to pack a bag in the event that you do need to go to hospital.

You will obviously need your typical overnight things like a few nighties, some underwear, toiletries, toothpaste and a toothbrush. It is also important to remember that you will need a substantial amount of sanitary protection as blood loss can continue for a few days after the birth, along with having some short term bladder weakness until you regain muscle function. Tampons are not permitted as the cervix may not close immediately after the birth and they can be dangerous. It is also important for the midwives to monitor your blood loss and they will need you to give them a rough guide on how much blood you are losing. You may want to buy a few pairs of disposable knickers for the first day or so following the birth as your own may become stained.

Also remember to take some breast pads even if you intend on bottle feeding as you may leak quite a lot of milk in the first few days.

It can be helpful to take in your own bath towel as they are usually softer than the ones the hospital issue and are a better size. Dressing gowns and slippers will be just as essential – hospital floors can be very cold!

You may not have thought of it but you might want some magazines and snacks for when you are in labour. If your pain relief is working well, you could find that the early stages of labour are quite long and relatively boring, leaving you feeling hungry and restless. Use this time to relax and build up your energy reserves.

Remember to take an outfit for coming home in. Although you will have lost most of your bump, you may still be unable to fit into your size 10 jeans for a few weeks. A tracksuit with an elasticated waist is ideal and comfortable.

You will need things for your baby as well as yourself. However, your baby really doesn't need much in the first few days. Two or three babygrows, some vests and a selection of booties and scratch mitts should be enough while you

'If your pain relief is working well, you may find that the early stages of labour are quite long and relatively boring, leaving you feeling hungry and restless. Use this time to relax and build up your energy reserves.'

are in hospital, but you will need a hat and a warm blanket when you go home (even in the summer). Also remember that if you are travelling by car, you will be unable to leave the hospital without a suitable and correctly fitted car seat.

It is helpful to take a baby towel for bathing your baby and a packet of nappies (even if you intend on using washable nappies at home) as some hospitals require you to purchase your own after the birth and hospital shops can be expensive.

It can be very helpful to make a note of who you want contacting when you go into labour or after the birth, and to keep a list of names and numbers in your bag. Along with this, you should keep plenty of change for the telephone and to cover any car park charges you may incur while at the hospital.

It is useful to have a notebook nearby that has all your useful telephone numbers in (it is handy to have the number for the hospital and local taxi service). You can also jot down the timings of your contractions, as your midwife will need to know when they started and how they are progressing.

'If you feel that you are losing fluid or are bleeding, it is always best to be assessed. Your membranes may be about to break or have already split.'

When to seek advice

You may start becoming more fretful about when labour will begin – every little ache, pain or difference can make you want to run to the phone and ring the hospital. Don't panic – you will almost definitely know when real labour has begun! However, there are certain times when you may want to seek advice.

If you feel that you are losing fluid or bleeding, it is always best to be assessed. Your membranes may be about to break or have already split.

If you suddenly feel that you are breathless, dizzy, having visual disturbances or as though you are swelling, please see your midwife or doctor urgently.

If you are used to feeling regular movements from the baby and they slow down in the last few weeks, don't worry as this is normal and many mums-to-be panic that there is something wrong. However, if you feel no movements at all for six hours or more then it may be best to see your midwife who can listen to your baby's heart rate and reassure you.

Braxton Hicks

Braxton Hicks contractions do not affect everyone and although they may occur, they can go unnoticed. They are essentially practice contractions and can vary in strength (from being very gentle to being similar to a proper contraction), and can often be mistaken for the first stages of labour.

They often become more noticeable as the pregnancy progresses and help the body prepare for the labour when it starts.

They don't usually last long and should subside with some calm, deep breathing. However, they can be alarming if you are not used to them, and it is always best to get yourself checked out if you are unsure. Be warned though, if you go to the hospital with every Braxton Hicks contraction you experience, you may be spending quite a lot of your time there!

Your emotions

Emotions during this last phase vary between women and while some feel that time is rushing by and they are not yet ready for the baby, others feel as though the time drags and they are getting fed up. Some days you may feel full of energy and highly motivated, and on other days you can feel as though you have no energy and are very emotional. This is all part of a normal pregnancy.

If you are planning on starting your maternity leave a few weeks before the birth, try and plan some time to enjoy yourself. Spend time with friends and family and allow them to pamper you.

It is also wise to use this time to take plenty of rest while you can and to mentally prepare yourself for the big lifestyle changes you are likely to face.

It is very common to feel nervous, scared and apprehensive as you prepare for the birth – very few women would say that they didn't feel these emotions at all. To ease your mind, spend some time reading books on the subject, discussing your feelings with friends and relatives, or browsing the Internet. Many websites can offer readers the chance to join networks where women can express their fears and find out more information on other women's experiences.

'It is very common to feel nervous, scared and apprehensive as you prepare for the birth. Very few women would say that they didn't feel these emotions at all.'

Many women find they are feeling less attractive and uncomfortable as their shape changes, and this can lead to a decrease in sexual desire. Discuss these feelings with your partner and try to find new ways of being intimate without having intercourse if you wish. Alternatively, some women find that their sexual appetite increases as the pregnancy progresses and, again, this is normal. As long as you are comfortable having sex then it is safe to do so. However, you may need to use different sexual positions as your bump may restrict you somewhat!

If you are feeling highly emotional or even depressed, remember that you are probably not sleeping too well and your hormones are all over the place, all of which contribute to a highly emotional state. If you are feeling very low a lot of the time, please speak to your doctor or midwife as there may be ways of easing your worries further.

Summing Up

The third trimester is the last stretch home before you meet your new arrival. By this stage your bump is probably very prominent and you may find that you have started to leak a little milk from your breasts.

At this stage most people are starting to buy baby items and are planning names and nursery designs. It is a good idea to pack your bag for hospital, whether you are having a hospital or home birth (just in case). Make sure everyone involved in the birthing process understands their role and has a contact number.

As the third trimester comes to an end, you will probably be a bit fed up, feel huge and are becoming a little anxious for the birth. Your emotions are also likely to be a little unpredictable. You should start thinking about maternity leave and putting your feet up for a few weeks before the labour comes.

Checklist

- Have I packed my bag?
- Do I have my partner's phone number for when labour begins?
- Do I know who to contact if something doesn't seem quite right?
- Do I need to read any more about labour or what to expect after the birth?

Chapter Six

Scans, Tests and Complications

Throughout your pregnancy you will be monitored closely by your obstetric team who are there to look after the needs of both you and your baby. The team may include doctors, midwives and sonographers, along with those who work in the laboratories analysing your samples.

You will be tested for different things during different stages of your pregnancy and while you should give your consent for these tests, you should know that they are only carried out to the benefit and wellbeing of you and your baby.

If at any time during a test you are unsure of why it is being carried out, or want to know more information, always feel free to ask your healthcare provider who will be happy to explain and answer your questions.

Routine tests and scans

The tests you will be offered may depend on your personal circumstances and past or current health status, although there are some tests that are offered routinely and are now seen as an integral part of the antenatal care.

The 12 week scan

The date of your 12 week scan is determined by the date of your last menstrual period. This scan has a very definite purpose: by taking exact measurements of your baby, for example from the top of the head to the base of the spine, the sonographer can determine how far along in your pregnancy you actually are

'Througout your pregnancy you will be monitored closely by your obstetric team who are there to look after the needs of both you and your baby.'

(you might not have exactly 12 weeks of gestation, but may be slightly under or even a few weeks over). The scan also gives you the first chance to see your baby moving around in its little home and to make sure there is a heart beat.

If you believe you may be further along than your last period dictates or have been bleeding, you may be offered this scan earlier to make sure everything is as it should be.

Many people are very excited about the first scan, while others are nervous and find the experience a little daunting. However, to make the scan more successful it is important to have a full bladder as this enables the sonographer to visualise the baby, womb and placenta in more detail and will provide a better result.

The 20 week scan

The 20 week scan takes a little longer and, as your baby is now more developed, much more detail can be examined. The sonographer will be able to check that the baby's growth is on target for its dates, can measure and observe the function of many of the major organs and even check for abnormalities such as a cleft palate or spinal deformities.

Urine and blood tests

Having your urine tested regularly throughout your pregnancy is very important and can tell your midwife many things. To you it may be a waste product that is best put down the toilet, but in actual fact your urine is a little mine of information.

At each scheduled (and often unscheduled) appointment you will be asked to provide a sample. This sample is tested for the presence of blood, protein and glucose among other things and may indicate early on that something needs assessing or treating.

For example, protein in your urine can indicate the first sign of pre-eclampsia, while the presence of blood may indicate that you have an infection. Both of these can be serious if left untreated.

Blood samples are taken for the same reason but offer different results. For example, your blood will tell the team what blood group you are, whether you are rhesus positive or negative and can be screened for the presence of infections such as hepatitis, HIV, your rubella status and whether you have any blood disorders.

3D and 4D scans

3D and 4D scans are relatively new to most centres and hospitals in the UK and are not routinely offered to all patients, with most having to arrange and pay for a private appointment.

They can be very comforting for parents as the baby can be seen in a lot more detail and the facial features may be seen. In a 4D scan the picture includes motion and you will be able to see how your baby actually moves in the womb. You may even be able to get a recording of this on DVD.

Having a 3D or 4D scan is not a necessary requirement of antenatal care. Healthcare providers are able to learn all they need from current scanning techniques, but many parents-to-be like to pay the (sometimes high) cost of being able to see a very detailed picture of their baby as he or she grows.

Amniocentesis

Amniocentesis is a specialised test that can help determine the chances of whether your baby will be born with any chromosomal disorders such as Down's syndrome. The test is not routinely offered as it isn't without risk, but may be considered by those who have had a blood test showing an increased chance or an indication on a scan. It may also be offered to those with a close family member who has Down's syndrome or if they are over the age of 35, as both of these factors increase the risk of a baby being born with a type of chromosomal disorder.

Your midwife will counsel you before having the test to make sure you are happy with your decision. Many couples decide that even if their baby is likely to have Down's, this will not affect the pregnancy or their relationship with the child. Others like to consider their options or prepare themselves more fully for bringing up a child with a chromosomal disorder.

'3D and 4D scans are relatively new to most centres and hospitals in the UK and are not routinely offered to all patients.'

The test is performed by taking a small sample of the amniotic fluid that surrounds the baby. This is done by inserting a very fine needle into your abdomen, guided by ultrasound scanning techniques. The baby will not be able to feel the test, but there is a slightly higher chance of miscarriage following the test than without it, which is why a great deal of thought must go into whether you have the assessment or not.

Complications

Gestational diabetes

'If you are told you have gestational diabetes, you will need to be more careful with your diet so that your blood sugars are not permitted to climb too high.'

Gestational diabetes is the name given to the type of diabetes that develops during pregnancy. In a normal human body enough insulin is produced to metabolise sugars in the bloodstream, but when you are pregnant your body must work harder. Some people (up to 15%) cannot carry this out effectively and their blood sugars remain high.

Often this type of diabetes will disappear after the birth, but during the pregnancy you will be monitored very closely. This is to help avoid any detrimental effects of having high blood sugars, such as having a bigger baby or a baby who needs more intensive care following the birth.

If you are told you have gestational diabetes, you will need to be more careful with your diet so that your blood sugars are not permitted to climb too high.

For more information on gestational diabetes, see *Diabetes – The Essential Guide* (Need2Know).

Ectopic pregnancy

An ectopic pregnancy is a potentially very serious condition. It occurs as the embryo implants into the wall of the fallopian tube instead of the womb lining. The embryo can continue to grow into a foetus which then becomes stunted by the narrow tubal structure. This can cause a lot of pain and there is a very serious risk of the tube bursting open, causing immense bleeding if not treated quickly.

If you are less than 12 weeks pregnant and experience vaginal bleeding or sharp pains in your lower abdomen, it is recommended that you seek urgent medical attention to be assessed for an ectopic pregnancy.

Hyperemesis gravidarum

Hyperemesis gravidarum means 'excessive vomiting during pregnancy'. It is common for women to experience frequent bouts of sickness in the early weeks, but this should lessen as the pregnancy progresses. For some, however, it doesn't and often gets worse. Normal morning sickness is nothing to worry about, but if you are losing weight and cannot keep anything down at all, day or night, then you should tell your midwife or GP who may be able to determine the cause and offer symptomatic relief.

It is not healthy to allow the sickness to continue as you may become dehydrated and exhausted, or you may even have an underlying condition that needs treating.

Pre-eclampsia

Pre-eclampsia is an extremely dangerous condition and your midwife will be observing you for signs of the illness at every appointment.

It is indicated by high blood pressure and unexpected or irregular swelling which occurs as fluid collects and is not being processed effectively by the body. As the fluid overloads your tissues and your blood pressure is not within a normal range, there is a chance that your baby is not getting all the oxygen and nutrients that it needs to grow and survive.

Those who are overweight and over 40 years of age, or are having a multiple birth, are at the most risk and will be monitored very closely.

Symphysis pubis

The symphysis pubis is the strong joint that keeps the front and back halves of your pelvis together. This tough joint allows very little movement between the two halves of the pelvis. However, in order to house and give birth to a baby, the body releases a chemical during pregnancy that relaxes the joint a little bit. Occasionally, extreme pain can result as the joint slackens, possibly because one half moves more and in opposition to the other. It is also possible that the joint can separate, leaving a very wide gap in your pelvic bones. This is called diastasis symphysis pubis which can be excruciatingly painful and may limit your movement.

Summing Up

Throughout your pregnancy you will be assessed and observed in many ways. This may mean you will need to provide urine and blood samples, allow your doctor or midwife to carry out a physical examination or undergo a series of scans or tests. These tests do not exist for any other reason than to make sure everything is progressing in the right way and that your health and that of your baby's is being maintained.

By carrying out these tests and examinations, your healthcare providers can detect any changes as soon as possible and can find out at the earliest opportunity whether any interventions are needed to protect or treat either you or your baby.

Chapter Seven

The Labour

For most women, the thought of labour induces panic and anxiety mixed with a lot of curiosity as to how they will manage it. While these issues can put people off reading and learning about labour, it is a very important part of the pregnancy and it is vital that women and their partners understand the first signs.

Although it can be a very long time between that very first twinge and actually having your baby, it is important that you listen to your body, understand what is happening and know how to manage it. Even more importantly, you must know when to seek help and advice and have your progress assessed.

Recognising labour

Every woman's labour will start at a different time with a unique symptom; some are very obvious, but others can disguise themselves as the normal effects of pregnancy. Some women may find that they suddenly feel a gush of warm fluid escaping from them followed by sudden and regular pains. Others feel nothing more than persistent backache for a few days and won't really believe that they are showing the first stages of labour.

The signs are highly variable in the early stages but, as time progresses and nature takes its course, the symptoms become more and more obvious.

In the days before your baby is born, you may find that you lose a mucous plug from your vagina. This is a jelly-like substance that often comes away in one piece, its purpose being to sit in the neck of the womb (the cervix) and protect your baby from infections. It is a very thick substance and difficult to penetrate.

'Every woman's labour will start at a different time with a unique symptom; some are very obvious, but others can disguise themselves as the normal effects of pregnancy.'

Though it doesn't happen for all women, one of the more common signs is when the waters break. This means that the sac of fluid that encases your baby has either started leaking slowly or has spontaneously ruptured.

If the membranes are leaking, the chances are you have had some fluid leaking slowly for the past day or so, but this can easily be mistaken for urine. If you suddenly feel a gush of water between your legs, your waters have probably broken. Make a note of the time and ring your midwifery unit or delivery suite. They will tell you to either come to hospital for assessment or will send your midwife to you if you have opted for a home birth.

It is important not to leave it too long before you seek medical advice as both you and your baby may be prone to infection after your waters have broken, and also because you may go into the next stage of labour very soon after. If at any time you feel you want to push, can feel something in your vagina or can feel a pressure on your cervix or in your vagina, please seek urgent medical help. These may be signs that something unsafe is occurring such as an imminent delivery, a prolapsed umbilical cord or perhaps your baby is not lying in a head down position. These will all need immediate professional help.

Whether your waters have broken or not, you will eventually find that you are feeling pain. This is unlike any pain you have experienced before but is often likened to very severe period pain. This is true to some degree but the pain incorporates your entire abdomen, instead of the usual lower pelvis and under-carriage as with period cramps.

The pain will build over a short time and may last overall for a minute or two (it will probably feel like forever) before subsiding until the next time. This stage of labour can continue for some time, so unless the pain is absolutely unbearable or you feel you want to push, spend 15 to 30 minutes timing your contractions to gauge how far apart they are and whether you can manage them without any form of relief.

Contractions can develop in strength and quicken over a very long time. For most women (especially those having their first baby), this is usually a chance for them to gather their thoughts and emotions and take things easy for a while.

'If your contractions are less than three minutes apart, you really can't manage the pain, your waters have broken or you feel an unbearable urge to push, you should ring your midwife immediately.'

Need2Know

Pain relief

Pain relief during labour is usually something that women start thinking about a lot earlier than the last trimester, as pain in labour is often the biggest fear that women have of being pregnant. For many this is true, while others find that the fear and anticipation is actually worse than the labour and delivery itself.

However, spending some time learning about the different types of pain relief that are available to you is a good idea. Not only does it help you decide on the type of birth you would like, but it can help the medical staff abide by your decisions as well. Also, you will have a greater understanding of how each type of pain relief will affect both you and the baby during labour and after the delivery.

It is not usually necessary to require pain relief in early labour as it can normally be tolerated if movement, relaxation and breathing techniques are used. In many hospitals, strong drugs for pain relief are only given when the pain is becoming totally unbearable.

Epidural

Epidurals are a common form of pain relief for women in labour. They involve the patient receiving an injection into the spinal region to numb the skin and surrounding area. This works very quickly and is followed by the insertion of a very fine tube into your back through which pain relieving drugs can be delivered. These drugs can last for around four hours after which they can be topped up if needed. The pain relief helps to numb the sensation of pain during contractions by interfering with the nerve supply and pain signals to the brain, but still allows the woman to feel touch and have the ability to push when required.

As epidurals are now so common, they are very accurate and often carry no risks or side effects. There is, however, the possibility of developing an 'epidural headache' in the hours or days following the procedure. Although this can be severe, it doesn't last for long.

The other possible disadvantage is the additional time of labour. This does not happen to all women who receive an epidural, but there is a chance your labour could slow down and your baby will take longer to arrive.

'Pain relief during labour is usually something that women start thinking about a lot earlier than the last trimester, as pain in labour is often the biggest fear that women have of being pregnant.'

As the drugs are given into your spinal area and not into the blood supply, there is little chance of them affecting the baby.

Most hospitals have an on-call doctor (anaesthetist) available 24 hours a day, though smaller units often can't offer this service. Make sure you discuss your plans for pain relief with your midwife as this may influence where you choose to have your baby.

Entonox

Otherwise known as 'gas and air', Entonox is by far the most common form of pain relief used by labouring women. It is a mixture of nitrous oxide and oxygen that women can inhale during episodes of intense pain to take the edge off. Gas and air is delivered by either a facemask or a mouthpiece. Many women find the mouthpiece most appropriate as it can be used to bite down on and is less restricting and claustrophobic than a facemask.

The greatest benefits of using Entonox include its speed of effectiveness, the fact that the patient can control the amount received, the duration it can be used for (and remains effective for) and because it carries no risk or effect to the baby.

All hospitals should have good supplies of Entonox, and many community midwives will be able to bring a portable canister to your home if you have opted for a home delivery. However, there is a small chance that the supply may run out if your labour is very lengthy.

The associated side effects can include feeling dizzy, feeling nauseous and having a dislike to the sensation the gas can give.

For those who have selected to have as little pain relief as possible, it is a good option for the last stages of labour that can be very painful.

Pethidine or diamorphine

Both pethidine and diamorphine are opiate drugs and are very strong. They must be used very carefully due to their strong effects and only qualified staff will be able to administer them.

They are given via an injection (usually in the leg) and work within 10 minutes, with very good effect for most. The biggest disadvantage is the chance of the drugs transferring to the baby and having a negative effect, such as causing breathing difficulties. There is an antidote for this effect but it may not work, and your baby could need help with ventilation shortly after the birth. Babies can also remain groggy and sleepy for the first few days. Due to these reasons, you may want to give extra thought to using either drug if you are having a home birth.

In some instances, the drugs can cause nausea and vomiting for the expectant mother and may leave a lasting effect for several hours after the delivery.

These drugs are not suitable to use in the very early stages of labour or as you are about to start pushing as they will not have had enough time to take full effect. They are of most use when the pain of the contractions is beginning to get overwhelming.

TENS machine

A TENS machine (transcutaneous electrical nerve stimulator) is a device often used for pain management, especially during labour. It works by sending electrical signals through your body that aim to stimulate the natural production of endorphins (pain relieving chemicals that we all produce naturally).

Using a TENS machine means that you are less likely to need injections or strong drugs, can remain more mobile during the labour and will experience no side effects.

They are very safe and involve placing two sticky pads on the mid-to-upper region of your spine (approximately where your bra strap is) which deliver the electrical pathways. By having the pads arranged in this location, they firstly encourage the natural release of endorphins which is nature's own pain relief, and secondly block pain signals to the brain. The mode of action depends on the frequency at which they are set.

If you would like to use this type of pain relief and wish to try it in the earlier stages of labour (as advised for this option), or are planning a home birth, please speak to your midwife. Your midwife will be able to tell you where the machine can be hired from, at what cost (if any) and how to use it correctly.

'Both pethidine and diamorphine are opiate drugs and are very strong. They must be used very carefully due to their strong effects and only qualified staff will be able to administer them.'

If you have a history of heart problems or epilepsy, it is essential that you also speak to your doctor as you may not be a suitable patient for this type of pain relief.

Choosing to have no pain relief

For some women (and men), the thought of having no pain relief at all during what is commonly considered to be one of life's most painful experiences, fills them with horror. For others, a positive mental attitude and having complete understanding and control of the labour, with no chance of side effects for either the mother or baby, is enough to make them plan to have no pain relief.

Of course, it is not always possible to endure the entire labour with no help at all and, very occasionally, a spinal or general anaesthetic may be needed if a caesarean section is required.

In the event that you decide to have no conventional pain relief at all, there are other options that can be explored that do not involve machines, drugs or any other medical paraphernalia and can work very well.

'In the event that you decide to have no conventional pain relief at all, there are other options that do not involve machines, drugs or any other medical paraphernalia and can work very well.'

Massage

Massage is a great way of controlling pain for many reasons and also offers a perfect opportunity to involve your partner in the labour. In fact, there is research available that shows that women who received massage during labour, whether it was from their partner, midwife or birthing partner, had shorter labours and managed better in the days and weeks following the delivery.

When a person is massaged, the action acts as a way of naturally stimulating endorphin production. These chemicals are something that we produce naturally to help make us feel better and block out pain signals.

It is an exceptionally good technique to learn during the pregnancy as a way of relaxing and taking it easy. Let your partner know which type of massage you like best so you are ready for when labour begins. Try choosing a few books on the subject, particularly those that relate to labour pain, or ask your midwife for advice.

Massage is also very good for those who are experiencing back pain during labour (often as a result of how the baby is laying in the womb) or for those who wish to have good control over their breathing.

It is useful to alternate the areas that are massaged; the back, shoulders, hands and feet are all good starting points.

Do remember that even if you have planned to have no conventional pain relief, the option will always be open to you if you feel that it is needed. No one can predict how you will cope during labour as it is a unique experience every time and one person's pain level is not going to be the same as anyone else's.

Using music to help you cope

It might not sound possible, but using music as a therapy may actually be very effective at reducing labour pain. Not only is it calming and lessens distress during the labour, it has been found to act as a distraction from the pain, improve the recovery following the delivery and seems to improve and encourage a good relationship between mother and baby.

Studies are continually proving how beneficial music can be to labouring mothers, and it has been found that the best types of music to use are those that make you feel calmer and less anxious.

If you plan on using music to help during your labour, please make sure you have the equipment to carry this out as many hospitals may not yet cater for it.

Where you can have your baby

Choosing where to have your baby is a decision most mothers-to-be make very easily and have very definite ideas about. However, others like to know a little about the benefits and disadvantages of each option before they make any plans.

Home births

Home births can have many advantages over hospital births and research continues to provide very good evidence of the benefits to both mother and baby.

It has been found that the mother has a much less traumatic experience of labour and birth if they have their baby in their own home. The atmosphere is relaxed, your partner can be fully involved, you can choose which room to deliver in (within reason) and there is less chance of either the mother or partner becoming anxious, which tends to speed up the labour and make the delivery easier. It is also likely that your delivering midwife will be someone who is already familiar to you and has built up a relationship with both you and your partner, whereas a hospital may provide many different midwives who are not familiar at all. Having a home birth means you may not need to make domestic arrangements, worry about making your way to the hospital or picking up an infection during your stay there.

'Home births can have many advantages over hospital births and research continues to provide very good evidence of the benefits to both mother and baby.'

There are, however, some disadvantages of choosing to have your baby at home. You may not have all pain relief options available to you, such as an epidural as this service cannot be offered in the community setting.

A home birth does not always guarantee that you will have no complications during the birth, and the emergency services are not just through the door as they would be in a hospital setting.

If you have had problems during your pregnancy, are carrying a multiple pregnancy or have any serious medical history, your midwife will probably explain why a hospital birth is safer for both you and your baby.

Midwife-led units

Having your baby in a clinical setting does not necessarily mean that you will need to travel miles to the nearest city hospital, as there are many midwife-led units up and down the country. These units are run by highly trained midwives and offer many of the services found in a hospital delivery suite. However, they may have no medical cover in the form of doctors.

These units offer the expertise of midwives in a relaxed environment, are often less 'medical' than traditional units and often cause less anxiety and stress, especially for those who feel intimidated by the hospital setting.

Many birthing centres or midwife-led units can offer other therapies and may be more accommodating to your requests than a traditional unit.

The disadvantages include not being able to receive an epidural as there are no anaesthetists and having to travel to a bigger unit or hospital if medical input is needed.

Hospital births

Many women are happy to have a hospital birth for many reasons, including the availability of pain relief, the provision for emergency input if required and because they simply feel it is the right thing to do.

Hospital births can be as comfortable as home births and many women have access to rocking chairs, birthing pools or other equipment if they want it, safe in the knowledge that there is help nearby if needed.

The disadvantages include being in an unfamiliar environment, finding the environment very clinical, noise from other patients and not being allowed to go home straight after the birth.

Choosing where to have your baby is a very personal choice, but it is still a good idea to pack a bag and know the way to the nearest hospital should you need to go in.

'Many birthing centres or midwife-led units can offer other therapies and may be more accommodating to your requests than a traditional unit.'

First stage labour explained

Labour is divided into three separate parts. This is mainly for healthcare professionals to refer to, but there are benefits to learning these stages so you know what to expect from the start of your labour to the very end.

First stage labour is the term given to the initial part of your labour when the pains begin. This is commonly the longest part of the labour and it is more beneficial for you to stay at home as long as possible during it. You will probably be more comfortable in your own surroundings and it saves a trip to the hospital where you will be assessed and often asked to return at a later stage of the labour when medical input is more likely to be required. The hospital will ask you to return home for a number of reasons, but mainly because of your own comfort – hospital surroundings can be very restricting. There is also a lack of available beds that cannot be used unnecessarily and your labour will progress more quickly and safely if you remain active, which is much easier in your own home than at hospital.

Your labour may begin with some period-like pain which progresses to a regular pattern of stronger and more frequent contractions. In the early stages they are often around 15 minutes apart and progress until one comes to an end and another begins within a minute or two. During these contractions your cervix should be gently dilating and softening, ready for the passage of the baby. This will also take some time – your cervix will need to dilate to a full 10 centimetres in order for the baby to pass through.

It is common during this time to need to change position frequently, pass urine or have a bowel movement. It is perfectly safe for you to move around during this stage as long as you don't feel like you need to push. Try not to let yourself get too tense or anxious as this may lengthen your experience and turn it into something negative, when in fact it should be embraced and remembered.

'Deep breathing and gentle massage during this time are great ways of relieving pain and discomfort, offering a welcome distraction from the contractions.'

Deep breathing and gentle massage during this time are great ways of relieving pain and discomfort, offering a welcome distraction from the contractions. It will help to relax your body and make the pushing stage easier.

Towards the end of the first stage of labour it is usual to want some form of pain relief, and when this time comes you should make your way to the hospital. When you have arrived, your midwife will assess your status and check your cervix to find out how far it has already dilated, followed by offering pain relief.

When your cervix has dilated to 10 centimetres and your contractions are coming faster and faster, you will be nearing the time when your body will tell you to push. This overwhelming urge cannot really be forced and you will know when you need to do it.

With the guidance of your midwife, you will progress to the second stage of labour.

Second stage labour explained

The second stage of labour is when the hard work begins and you must deliver your baby into the world. When your cervix has fully dilated, your baby will be pushing itself down the birth canal. This feels very heavy in your lower pelvis and it cannot be held back. Each contraction will lower the baby further into the birth canal and at the end of the contraction he or she may ease back a little, but this is natural.

Your midwife will tell you exactly when to push, how long for and when to stop. If everything is going without any problem, your midwife will tell you when to ease off a little with the pushing. This is so your vaginal skin and the surrounding area have time to expand gently and to minimise the risk of you suffering a tear. When the next contraction comes, you can resume pushing. If your baby is head down, your midwife may invite you to place your hand to your vagina if you want to feel the baby's head crowning. As this area stretches to accommodate the baby's head, you may find that it stings and makes you want to stop, but reassure yourself that the more you can bear it, the quicker your baby will be born.

Once your baby's head is delivered, the hardest part is done and it often only takes a few more pushes to deliver the rest of the baby. After this, you can relax for a while and enjoy every second of meeting your new son or daughter. Make this time special by having your baby lay on your naked skin; this is called skin-to-skin contact and midwives all around the world advise that this is one of the best ways to bond with your baby, calm a newborn and successfully instigate breastfeeding.

Third stage labour explained

The third stage of labour is the term used to describe the delivery of the placenta. This can be an assisted process whereby you are given an injection into your thigh as the baby is born that helps the body eject the placenta, or it can be a natural delivery.

A natural delivery of the placenta takes longer but means that you won't have the injection. Your womb must continue contracting (though obviously not to the same degree as before) and can take up to an hour to expel the placenta.

This process may be advanced by the instigation of breastfeeding which naturally causes gentle contractions of the womb.

In very few cases, the placenta does not come away completely or even not at all (more common in smokers) and it may need to be removed manually. In this instance you may need an operation.

Types of birth

'Once your baby's head is delivered, the hardest part is done and it often only takes a few more pushes to deliver the rest of the baby.'

Although the media often portrays childbirth as being in agony followed by some pushing in a hospital bed, this may not be the type of birth that you experience. Not only may you have some input into the birthing process, but nature may dictate that further assistance is needed to guarantee the health and safety of both you and your baby.

Normal delivery

A normal delivery is the name given to those births that have not required any medical intervention other than perhaps an episiotomy (a small incision made between the vagina and anus so there is more space for the baby to pass through). Your delivery will be described as normal if your labour progresses without any major complications and the baby is born vaginally. The birth is still referred to as a normal delivery if your waters are broken for you or you are induced.

You can decide while you are in labour which form of third stage you would like. Your midwife will discuss this with you if you haven't decided.

Water birth

Planning a water birth is usually something that either appeals to women or doesn't at all. If you are thinking of trying a water birth, it is important to find out what facilities are available in your local hospital or community services.

Some areas offer water pools as an option for home births and largely support this choice, whereas other places cannot offer the same. Likewise, your local hospital or birthing centre may be very well geared up for providing a pool, whereas others have no such facilities.

You must speak at length to your midwife about a water birth and decide whether you want to deliver in the pool itself or whether you would prefer to use the pool while in the first stage of labour and then get out when you want to push.

Giving birth in a pool does not pose any risk to your baby as he or she will not start to breathe until their body is out of the water.

The water is usually warm and can help you relax, and is also a great way of involving your partner in the birthing process.

Assisted delivery

Babies that are born using either forceps or ventouse are said to have had an assisted delivery. This means that although the baby has been born vaginally, specialist instruments have been used to help the safe delivery of the baby. These may be needed if your baby is not progressing through the vagina but has already come some of the way, if he or she is getting distressed or because you are too exhausted to continue.

If forceps are used, large steel-cupped spoons are placed around the baby's head so that it can be gently pulled or guided down the remainder of the canal.

A ventouse delivery means that a small suction cup is placed on the baby's head and a vacuum process is used to perform a similar action.

During each of these procedures you may have to place your legs in stirrups so that the doctor or midwife has appropriate access to the baby.

'Giving birth in a pool does not pose any risk to your baby as he or she will not start to breathe until their body is out of the water.'

Caesarean sections

A caesarean section involves making a surgical incision into your bikini line through to your womb and the baby. The procedure is carried out by obstetric surgeons and can be done using a general anaesthetic, a spinal anaesthetic or by having your existing epidural 'topped-up'.

Many women request a caesarean section, although there may be some areas that don't advise this form of delivery unless it is absolutely necessary for the health and safety of the mother and child.

For many women, a caesarean section will be advised before the labour has even begun. This can be for a number of reasons: perhaps the baby is very large, you may not have perfect health or the baby may be lying in the breech position. In these instances the date of the delivery is planned in advance so you can organise things around this time. This is also good for your birthing partner who can make the appropriate arrangements too.

In some instances the operation may be performed as an emergency. This may be because the labour is not progressing, the baby is distressed, you are losing too much blood, the cord has delivered before the baby or you are having a multiple birth.

If the operation is carried out as a dire emergency, it is important to remember that it is being performed for the health of both you and your baby – and sometimes time is of the essence.

If you have a caesarean section, you will find that you might have a urinary catheter afterwards, along with drips and wound drains. These are nothing to worry about and are often given as a routine safety issue.

Unless you are having your operation under a general anaesthetic, your partner or birthing partner may accompany you to the delivery room and sit with you during the procedure. After the baby is born, he or she will be checked over by the midwife or doctor, after which you will be able to see your baby.

It is not uncommon for babies born by caesarean section to need a little bit of oxygen or oral suctioning after the birth. Try not to be too alarmed if this occurs.

Episiotomies and vaginal tears

If you have a normal vaginal delivery (with or without the use of forceps or ventouse), there is a chance that your perineum (the area between your vagina and rectum) can become damaged.

If the midwife can observe the area, guide you through the pushing stage of labour or can predict that a tear is likely, an episiotomy can be performed. This means local anaesthetic is used and the area is numbed and a careful cut is made. Although this may sound horrific, it can significantly reduce the complications (short and long term) of suffering a natural tear. Following the delivery, the area is sewn up using absorbable sutures. After having an episiotomy, most women find they have no problems with the healing or any long term issues.

If, however, the baby progresses very quickly, gets stuck half way out, turns during the delivery or you do not follow the pushing instructions given by your midwife, there is a chance you may tear. A minor tear can sometimes heal by itself but more serious tears may involve several layers of tissue and will need surgically repairing.

'It is not uncommon for babies born by caesarean section to need a little bit of oxygen or oral suctioning after the birth. Try not to be too alarmed if this occurs.'

Summing Up

When your baby is ready to make an entrance into the world, you will need to make a few decisions including the type of pain relief you prefer, where you would most like to have your baby and who you want with you during the labour.

Occasionally, nature will dictate some of your choices but it can be very helpful to have a plan so that the doctors, nurses and midwives can do their best to carry out your preferences.

Labour can begin at any time and will be a unique experience for every woman and their partner. Your body and baby may take several hours to progress to the delivery, while others may have a speedy labour and give birth soon after the first pain.

In some circumstances, you may need assistance delivering your baby safely. This may result in an episiotomy, using suction or forceps or even a caesarean section. If this is the case, it is helpful to try and comply as much as possible as this will ensure the overall health and safety of both you and the baby.

Checklist

- Will I know when labour has begun?
- Do I know who to contact and when?
- Is my bag ready?
- Do I know where the nearest hospital or birthing centre is?
- Have I got change for the telephone?
- Are my medical notes packed in my bag?
- Have I had a think about pain relief and know which methods I would prefer?

Chapter Eight

The First Few Days

Congratulations on becoming a parent. You have grown and looked after your baby inside you, and now he or she has made their arrival. But what happens next?

Your body

It is very common to feel physically exhausted in the first few days but this is often accompanied by feelings of elation. Your body has accomplished something fantastic and your mind is full of taking in the sight and smell of your little one. The emotions and tiredness can compete, leaving you feeling a little strange.

It is also common to feel slightly anxious about whether you will know how to look after a baby and what happens next, but also a sense of anti-climax as you realise that for the first few days and weeks you are at someone else's beck and call. Suddenly the reality has hit.

In the days after the birth, though for some it happens very quickly, your breasts should start producing milk, often in great quantities. You may find that even the sound of your baby crying is enough to instigate the flow of milk and you must feed him or her immediately. Others may find that though they want to breastfeed, their milk is not as apparent; this is nothing to worry about and your midwife will help you achieve successful breastfeeding, although a little patience and perseverance may be needed.

If you choose to breastfeed, you will probably find that your womb contracts when the baby is attached to the breast; this is a totally natural occurrence and happens because of hormones being released by the breastfeeding process, but it can be quite painful until you are used to it.

'Your body has accomplished something fantastic and your mind is full of taking in the sight and smell of your little one. The emotions and tiredness can compete, leaving you feeling a little strange.'

Passing urine more frequently is usual and nothing to become anxious about as it is simply your body expelling all of the fluid it has accumulated during the past few months. You will find your weight decreases steadily for a few days and you appear less swollen and bloated than before. It may, however, mean that you pass urine without being totally aware of it as your body is still quite numb and stretched from the birth. This is not usually permanent and should settle after a few weeks or months.

It is also likely that passing urine will sting for the first few times as your vagina and vulva are stretched, bruised and traumatised. It may help to try and pass urine in the bath or shower for the first few times to ease the discomfort.

Bleeding happens to everyone who has had a vaginal delivery and to most that have had a caesarean section. This is because the inside of your womb does not need to be as thick and protective as it had been when it housed your baby. The excessive tissue and cells will gradually be expelled through your vagina and will be quite red and heavy for the first couple of days, or even a week, but will lose colour and amount over time. Your midwife will keep a log of your physical progress and will ask you about your blood loss, so don't be afraid to be graphic; they are used to it and need the information.

After giving birth, your body contains many hormones at unusual levels and this can cause changes to your hair and skin. You may find your skin becomes more dry or greasy and that you are losing a lot of hair. This will settle down as your hormone levels return to normal and your monthly cycle returns.

Feeding your baby

Many women know exactly how they plan to feed their baby long before the birth, and stick to these plans without giving it much thought. But it can be very helpful to know a little about each method of feeding so that you are sure you are making the best decision for both you and your baby.

Breastfeeding

The old saying 'breast is best' exists for a reason. Mammals naturally produce breast milk to give their babies everything they need to achieve the best state of health. The benefits of breastfeeding are not just reaped in the early years as they can be seen in the future too.

The physical and nutritional benefits include protection against infections and illnesses as the breast milk contains many antibodies. These antibodies can help to protect your baby from ear, chest and gastro-intestinal related complaints.

Apart from the nutritional benefits of breast milk, there are many other advantages of feeding your baby this way. Firstly, there will be no need to stagger down the stairs at three in the morning to make a bottle as you can simply sit on the edge of your bed or even lay down with your baby (as long as you don't fall asleep!). Secondly, compared to bottle fed babies, your baby will need less winding and is less likely to suffer from colic or other problems with trapped wind. Thirdly, there is the advantage of establishing a very close bond with your new baby as the closeness is unique, and often you will find that you are both happy to spend the feed gazing into each other's eyes and making those first weeks and months extra special.

Breastfed babies also seem to sleep better as they are more content and satisfied after the feed. In fact, they can appear to be drunk after the feed, they are that happy! There is even evidence to suggest that breastfed babies do better in school and are less likely to suffer with obesity and weight gain in later life.

Along with all these benefits, there are some more slightly selfish, but nevertheless important, facts that should be remembered. Unless you plan to express your breast milk, you will have no reason to sterilise equipment. Also, there is significant evidence that nursing mothers are protected from breast and ovarian cancers in the long term. You are also more likely to regain a slender figure as breastfeeding can burn off many calories.

'Mammals naturally produce breast milk to give their babies everything they need to achieve the best state of health.'

What happens?

When breastfeeding is commenced, the fluid is watery and a yellow colour; this is called colostrum and lasts for a few days. After this, your breast milk should start appearing.

When a baby initiates a feed, they receive the foremilk first which is the equivalent of having a drink before your meal or having soup as a starter. The hindmilk is then released which fills your baby and gives all the nutrients.

How to breastfeed

'The best way to ensure successful breastfeeding is to have skin-to-skin contact straight after the delivery if you can.'

The best way to ensure successful breastfeeding is to have skin-to-skin contact straight after the delivery if you can. This means that the baby is laid on your bare chest as soon as he or she is born. Babies have a natural ability to suckle and will route for your breast as a natural reaction. Allow your baby to find his or her way to the nipple, then gently assist them in latching on. You can practise a successful 'latch' by gently sucking on the fleshy area of the back of your hand as opposed to sucking the end of your finger. When your baby is sucking properly, he or she should have taken most of your areola (the area around the nipple) into the mouth and not just the nipple. He or she should also be able to breathe comfortably and not have to adjust in order to take a breath. If you put your nipple to the baby's nose, this will encourage them to tip his or her head back. You can then point the nipple to the roof of the mouth and let them latch on this way.

When breastfeeding, always bring the baby towards you. Try not to lean or hunch over as this will result in a poor technique, as well as giving you very severe backache!

Your arm should be supporting the full length of the baby, keeping its body in line with yours. Sometimes a pillow behind you, or even supporting your arm, can help if your baby takes a long time to feed.

When you are breastfeeding, it is currently advocated that you feed on demand and let your baby dictate when he or she needs another feed.

Mastitis

Mastitis is a condition that commonly affects breastfeeding mothers. It is the name given when the breast itself becomes inflamed. This can cause hardness, swelling, redness and pain. It can affect both breasts, but this is fairly unusual.

It occurs in breastfeeding mothers because either the breast is not being fully emptied or there is a blockage in the milk ducts.

The condition can sometimes be avoided by making sure you alternate the breasts that you use for feeding and by trying to make sure the breast is emptied at each feed. If your baby doesn't empty the breast, it may be useful to learn how to express the rest of the breast milk yourself by hand.

Massage can help relieve the symptoms, along with continuing to breastfeed in order to resolve the problem. Speak to your midwife or GP if symptoms persist.

Bottle feeding

Choosing to bottle feed may be something that you have considered since the beginning, but for some the choice is made for them. Not all women can successfully breastfeed for many reasons and this drives them to use formula milks. Although the advice is to breastfeed and no one would disagree with that, there are some benefits to bottle feeding that may be enough to ease the blow or make the decision.

The benefits and disadvantages

The biggest advantage of bottle feeding is the ability to share the feeding regime with someone else. This is a great way of involving your partner or family members in helping with the baby and allows you some time alone. Perhaps you could share the night feeds if your partner is taking paternity leave while you recover from the labour, or maybe grandparents can come round and give you time to have a bath.

'Although the advice is to breastfeed and no one would disagree with that, there are some benefits to bottle feeding that may be enough to ease the blow or make the decision.'

Bottle feeding also allows you the advantage of knowing exactly how much your baby is taking in one feed, something that may be quite difficult with breastfeeding.

Many people are also unaware that bottle fed babies tend to be less demanding with their feeds, as the formula takes longer to digest and thus keeps them full for longer. This can be very appealing if you have a busy life and will find it hard to sustain a very demanding baby.

'If you are going to bottle feed, it is essential to wash and sterilise the bottles, rings and teats properly to protect your baby from digesting old remnants of milky deposits, which can make them very poorly.'

There are, however, some disadvantages to bottle feeding that may dissuade you. The sucking action needed to drink from the teat may cause your baby to take in more air with their milk, which may give them an upset tummy or trapped wind. This can be very distressing for both you and your baby and may take a while to resolve. There is also a higher chance of your baby getting ear and chest infections, and being less protected against illnesses such as asthma in later life.

Another disadvantage is the need for sterilising. Sterilising equipment can be expensive and takes up a lot of time until you get used to it. The type of steriliser you choose will determine the amount of time the action takes. You can also only make up a few bottles of water at one time which can be kept in the fridge once cooled, and the feed made up and warmed when needed. This can be very limiting if you need to travel, for example.

If you are going to bottle feed, it is essential to wash and sterilise the bottles, rings and teats properly to protect your baby from digesting old remnants of milky deposits, which can make them very poorly. It's vital that you make up the feeds to the exact specifications described on the tin, making sure they are not too strong or too dilute, which can also make your baby ill very quickly.

Once you have decided to bottle feed your baby, it is very difficult (and sometimes impossible) to change to breastfeeding, so it is important to make a fully informed decision and understand that the choice is probably permanent.

Sterilising and equipment

It is very important that you sterilise all of your baby's bottles, rings and teats in the first six to 12 months of life. When babies are born, their immune systems are very immature, leaving them susceptible to many bacterial and viral infections. Making sure that you remove any pathogens or germs from the feeding equipment by sterilising can lessen this risk.

There are several types of sterilising equipment on the market, ranging from cold water sterilisation to microwaveable or steam sterilising.

When you are making the decision on the type of equipment you would like, make sure you read all the instructions on the packaging so that you are fully aware and capable of how to do it. If you need any assistance, please speak to your midwife who can provide all the information you need.

Sleeping

Trying to find time to sleep with a baby is always a hot topic. You may think that babies sleep all the time and you won't have any problems. However, a baby who is not settled at night or cannot easily be comforted after a feed may cry for several hours with no let up. Over a few weeks this can be physically and mentally draining.

Try to remember that your baby is only going to be this small and dependent for a few months and things will improve.

Most newborns sleep a lot during the day and this is the time when you can catch up on your own sleep. You may find that you want to use this time to catch up on housework, phone calls or seeing friends, but these things can wait; you have the rest of your life to clean the house. If your friends and family want to help out, why not ask them to take the baby for a walk for an hour when he or she is awake so that you can do your chores, leaving you to have a sleep with the baby when they return?

For the first few months, it is probably good advice to let your baby sleep in the same room as you, providing it is warm, safe and free from cigarette smoke. If the baby's crib or Moses' basket is near your bed, you can reach him or her and comfort them very easily. It is also good for feeding as you can gently lay your baby back down after a night feed and know that they will remain asleep.

Don't be tempted to put your baby in your bed as there are huge risks associated with this, such as suffocation, becoming too hot, rolling out or being rolled on by you or your partner. It may be comforting to let them lay there while they are taking a feed but they really should get used to sleeping alone.

When your baby is in his or her crib, there is no need to wrap them up so much that they end up sweating. If you have a reasonably warm house, there will be no need to use hats as your baby uses the head to keep their temperature even. A vest, babygrow and a nice warm blanket are enough.

A sleeping baby will probably feel as though they have cool hands and feet, but this is totally normal as they reserve their body heat for their vital organs. Don't be tempted to give them too many covers, but if they feel generally cold all over, this indicates that another layer is needed.

'A baby should be laid on his or her back with their arms free and their feet an inch or two away from the bottom of the crib.'

Make sure all bedding is tucked in so that the baby cannot pull it over their face, and ensure that you place your baby at the bottom of the crib so there is no chance of them wriggling under the covers and suffocating. A baby should be laid on his or her back with their arms free and their feet an inch or two away from the bottom of the crib.

Dietary issues

Regardless of whether you are bottle feeding or breastfeeding your baby, there is no need to give them anything else in the first few weeks, after which only cooled, boiled water may be offered as an alternative (this is especially important if they are not well). Occasionally, relatives will want to spoil the baby and offer them juice or something similar, but you must insist that they are not to be given it. Aside from the risk of poisoning or catching an infection, a baby's digestion and urinary system cannot cope with anything else.

As for you, you must make sure you eat regularly in order to retain energy for looking after your little one. Most importantly, if you are breastfeeding you should drink double the amount of liquid you normally would as you are losing a lot of fluid during every feed. It can be useful to take a small snack and a drink every time your baby feeds to make sure you stay hydrated and energised.

Nappies

There are two choices when it comes to nappies: disposable or re-useable. Years ago there was no such choice and families managed just fine with terry towelling nappies and were used to washing and drying them. Modern society has given us the creation of disposable nappies and, as convenient as they are, they do cause some problems. The main disadvantage of disposable nappies is the cost; over a year several hundreds of pounds will be spent on nappies, and some children continue to need them until they are three or four, taking the cost into thousands. There is also the environmental issue to be aware of – they take several years to biodegrade and contribute to many overflowing landfill sites around the world.

If you would like to consider using washable nappies, speak to your midwife as there is likely to be a nappy service in your area. This means that soiled nappies are collected and freshly laundered ones are dropped off at a fraction of the cost of disposable nappies. You may need to be taught by a professional how to put on and remove the nappy, but, once taught, this skill is not forgotten.

Your baby's needs

In actual fact, your baby doesn't have too many needs in the first few months and will be happy to be kept clean, warm, fed and loved. However, you may still be slightly unsure of exactly what you need to buy either before or just after the birth.

'Your baby doesn't have too many needs in the first few months and will be happy to be kept clean, warm, fed and loved.'

Clothes

There is no need to rush out and buy your baby a full wardrobe as soon as they are born; they grow out of them very quickly. For the first few days a selection of vests and babygrows will be enough. Make sure there is a clean one for every day and after a bath, with a few spare in case of vomiting or nappy leaks. You may want to buy a few outfits for days out, along with some scratch mitts and hats, and a snowsuit or thick blanket for travelling out of the home, but this should be enough. It is likely that you will be given clothes as gifts anyway and will end up having plenty.

Although many shops sell soft shoes for newborns, these offer no purpose than to look nice and are not necessary. In fact, many foot specialists recommend that babies do not wear shoes in the first year or until they are walking as their foot growth could be restricted, hindering their development.

Winding

Winding your baby is important; trapped gas can cause a lot of discomfort and greatly distresses your baby, causing him or her to cry as they cannot get comfortable.

It is necessary to wind your baby during and after a feed. This can be done by sitting them in an upright position, supporting their head, neck and chin with one hand and gently rubbing or patting their back with the other. You can also place them to your shoulder if this does not work. Burps may be small and often or come out in one big sound, leaving your baby with room to take a little more feed or to sleep comfortably. After a month or two, you will be more able to bring their wind up with less encouragement.

If you are having problems with winding, speak to your midwife or health visitor. They may suggest a change in the type of bottle you are using or a suitable remedy which can normally be purchased in general shops, chemists or supermarkets.

Naming your baby

There are many things to think about when deciding on your baby's name. It is worth considering how it will sound with their surname, if it can be shortened, what nicknames might arise from it, if there are any particular family names you would like to use and whether you and your partner both agree.

When the baby is first born and is in hospital, it is normal for the midwives to simply call them after your surname, for example 'female infant Johnson'. You do not have to decide straightaway and may find that the name you had planned all along simply doesn't suit your newborn. As long as you have a name in mind when you register the birth, you will be fine.

Registering your baby

Registering your baby is a legal requirement and must be done within six weeks of the birth. Make an appointment with your nearest registry office to ensure you register within the allotted time.

Your midwife will give you a form when the baby is born that must be kept safe until you go to register. Either parent can register the baby if you are married, but if you are not you must both go together and sign the form in agreement.

The details needed include the full names of you, your partner (if they are registering also) and the baby, as well as their sex and date and place of birth. This information is recorded on a legal document which is then signed by all parties. You will be a given a copy and the registrar will keep a copy. Additional copies may be ordered at a cost.

'Registering your baby is a legal requirement and must be done within six weeks of the birth. Make an appointment with your nearest registry office to ensure you register within the allotted time.'

Your emotions

Your emotions are likely to be very unpredictable for the first few days; your body is surging with hormones and all of a sudden you are an adult with a child who you are totally responsible for. You are likely to be elated, overwhelmed, underwhelmed and quite astounded by the feelings you have for your child and partner.

The baby blues

Experts now agree that the baby blues is something experienced by over half of all new mothers. It is assumed that this happens as a response to the sudden change in hormones, anxiety, tiredness and because the pregnancy is now over and a sense of anti-climax kicks in.

The baby blues can start straight after delivery or within a day or so, and may result in you feeling irritable, weepy, desolate, lonely and uncertain. As your hormones settle, your mood should improve and you will feel more like you had anticipated you would before the birth. If, however, your feelings and emotions do not improve and you continue to feel negative, you may be developing postnatal depression which is altogether more serious.

'Postnatal depression is thought to affect up to 10% of all new mothers and is now a recognised condition.'

Postnatal depression

Postnatal depression is thought to affect up to 10% of all new mothers and is now a recognised condition.

It can occur for a specific reason but often the actual cause remains unknown. It can creep up very slowly, with many individuals not realising they are feeling low, upset, irritable or anxious, and often those around them are the first to pick up on the problem.

Finding friends who have just had babies, or speaking to existing friends and family, may be enough to help you vent your feelings and get some reassurance that you are managing perfectly well. But if the feelings continue or get worse, you must seek help.

Asking for help

There are several reasons why women do not ask for help with their postnatal depression. Perhaps they do not realise they have it and believe that this is how life is going to be from now on. They often feel guilty about not enjoying motherhood but don't want to admit it for fear of being told they cannot look after their baby. Maybe they are scared of admitting that being a parent isn't exactly as they'd imagined. Whatever the reason, it is essential to ask for help as these negative feelings can grow worse and worse, eventually affecting your relationship with your baby and partner, your self-esteem and your self-worth. They may even pose a risk to either you or your baby.

Your GP or health visitor are the best people to seek advice from regarding postnatal depression. The depression occurs as a result of biological and environmental factors that are out of your control, so the diagnosis is definitely not a sign of failure. You may or may not need medication to help you through this time as there are many other therapies that can be very useful, but it is vital that you seek help before your depression escalates.

Going it alone – single parents

Bringing a child into the world alone may be something you have done by choice or have had decided for you. Either way, this may make you more determined to be the best parent you possibly can, and can motivate you to keep at it. Fortunately, there are several support groups and agencies that assist single parents in raising their children and there is no reason in the world why you shouldn't join them.

It is hard going it alone. Managing night-feeds, finances and a social life can be very difficult, but you will reap all the benefits once your child is more grown-up. Enjoy every minute and find comfort in the fact that the child rearing is all on your terms; there will be no arguments around the child and you can bring him or her up as you choose.

Friends and family can be extremely valuable to single parents, especially when sharing the experience of pregnancy, childbirth and watching your child reach their landmarks. But don't be afraid to ask them for help when things are tough or when you know you will need extra support.

If you are a single parent, make sure you know your rights and financial arrangements and make use of as many external support networks as you feel you need to.

For more information on coping on your own, please refer to *Single Parents – The Essential Guide* (Need2Know).

'There are several support groups and agencies that assist single parents in raising their children and there is no reason in the world why you shouldn't join them.'

Summing Up

Once the pregnancy is over and your baby has been born, you will need a few days to settle in with your little one and get to know each other. Some couples find this time an extremely calm and peaceful experience and embrace it positively, while others may find that the labour has left them too tired or with a feeling of anti-climax. Give yourself time to adjust to being a parent and take one day at a time; there is no rush – your baby will be with you for a long time yet!

'If you are a single parent, make sure you know your rights and financial arrangements and make use of as many external support networks as you feel you need to.'

You may worry that your baby hasn't enough clothes, toys or other baby things, but there really is no need to worry about this as newborns need a small selection of clothes (mainly babygrows) and don't play with toys for a few months yet. As long as your baby is fed, warm, clean and loved, he or she will have everything they need.

If, however, you really feel as though you are going to struggle and cannot cope, it is absolutely vital that you tell your midwife or health visitor. They will be able to provide many strategies for helping you cope and will have faced this problem before. The worst thing to do is keep it all to yourself, letting the feelings grow.

Chapter Nine

Multiple Births

Finding out you are pregnant is both exhilarating and worrying, but to then find out you are having more than one baby at the same time can be quite alarming. You may have found out early on, often at a scan, that twins, triplets or more are on their way. For a very small number of cases, the subsequent baby or babies are a complete surprise.

Your chances of having a multiple birth are increased if there is a family history of twins or more on the mother's side of the family or if you have had fertility treatment to conceive.

Is it different?

You will find that you will need to attend more appointments and scans when you are expecting twins or more. It is also more likely that you will be put directly under the care of a doctor, when those with a single and healthy pregnancy will not need to be. This means that you may have to attend a hospital appointment instead of being seen by your midwife at home or in his or her clinic.

You can also expect to be screened more frequently for conditions such as pre-eclampsia and diabetes, which are more common in a multiple pregnancy.

With regards to your growing abdomen, you may be surprised at how much it grows and stretches to accommodate your brood. Twins and triplets can grow to 35-37 weeks of gestation, by which time you will probably be extremely big and less able to get around comfortably.

'Your chances of having a multiple birth are increased if there is a family history of twins or more on the mother's side of the family or if you have had fertility treatment to conceive.'

You may also find that each baby has a different sleeping pattern and moves in a different way to the other/s, giving you the opportunity to get to know each baby a little more each day and discover their personality, as small as they may be.

It is unlikely that you will reach 40 weeks of gestation. Doctors expect a twin pregnancy to achieve around 37 weeks which is considered full term for a multiple pregnancy. If you deliver at this stage, you can expect your babies to be slightly smaller than the average, but they may still reach around 5lb in weight. Sometimes one twin or triplet can be a lot larger than the other, indicating that he or she received the most nutrients and blood flow while in the womb. Don't worry – the other baby will soon catch up!

'People have always been having multiple births and, with the advances in medical technology, it is safer now than it has ever been.'

How do they happen?

There are two reasons why multiple births occur. Firstly, one egg is fertilised and then splits into two or more embryos. These then grow into identical offspring (usually twins, occasionally triplets). The second form of multiple birth happens when more than one egg is fertilised at the same time, resulting in non-identical siblings. Although it is extremely rare, it is possible to find that both scenarios have occurred and both identical and non-identical siblings are born!

There has been a steady increase in those having multiple births in recent years. This can largely be attributed to the use of fertility treatments and IVF, as these greatly increase the chances of a multiple conception. The fact that many women are leaving motherhood to their thirties and forties also increases the risk.

However, people have always been having multiple births and, with the advances in medical technology, it is safer now than it has ever been.

Giving birth to more than one baby

Giving birth to more than one baby at a time can be extremely frightening for the mother. Not only will there be the added stress on her body during the pregnancy, but two babies (or more) need delivering and there's the thoughts of 'how will I cope?' after the birth.

There are some benefits to having more than one baby at the same time, though. The children will always have a playmate, you may not feel the need to have any future pregnancies, you only need to take one lot of maternity leave and, of course, you only have to look after a newborn once as it is doubled up!

When the actual delivery of the babies come, you may have been advised to have an elective caesarean section. This can be beneficial for you as the date of delivery can be planned in advance and your babies can be delivered in a controlled environment, before they grow too big for your body. If, however, you are planning a vaginal delivery, it is more likely that you will go into spontaneous labour earlier than women carrying just one.

The first baby will progress with a normal labour, with the second coming within a few minutes, leaving you enough time to get your breath back before you have to do it again.

Coping with a multiple birth

The mere sight of seeing two heart beats on the scanner may be enough to send you into a panic, but remember, people do cope and are actually very grateful that they have been blessed with more than one baby at a time.

The prospect of having to give birth more than once at the same time, coping with feeds, costs, sleeping arrangements, clothes and crying can be very daunting. But with help and organisation, it is possible. When your routine is established, you will see the benefits of having more than one baby at the same time.

Having a multiple birth means you will be monitored a lot closer than those carrying just one baby. There are several reasons for this but ultimately the goal is to protect both you and your babies from any complications, and to spot any problems early on so they can be dealt with before they become a risk.

There are many support groups available to those with twins, triplets or more, and you should join these and seek advice when you need it. It is likely that there will be some additional resources and help in your area, so just ask your midwife or health visitor for more information.

Risks of having a multiple birth

Having a multiple birth does carry the same risks as carrying one baby, but there are some added factors that will be monitored. Not only is there the risk of delivering earlier than a woman carrying a single pregnancy, but the process may also be more complicated.

There is a higher chance of developing pre-eclampsia, gestational diabetes and finding that your babies don't have the resources or room to develop as strongly as a single baby would. However, you will be assessed and monitored for all complications and any slight variance in your health will be acted upon. All you need to do is make sure you follow any advice given.

Summing Up

Having more than one baby at a time can be a frightening proposition but something that parents all over the world have faced and seem to cope very well with. It is true that your work may be cut out in the first couple of years, but there are so many advantages that can help soften the harshness of the difficult times.

You will be monitored very closely and may well go into labour at an earlier stage, but doctors do expect this and will make the appropriate provisions.

Making sure you are organised is very important when having more than one baby, especially during feeding, changing and when instigating a sleeping routine, but finding your own way of doing things will come eventually.

'Making sure you are organised is very important when having more than one baby, especially during feeding, changing and when instigating a sleeping routine, but finding your own way of doing things will come eventually.'

Chapter Ten

Maternity Leave and Benefits

For some women, their career and future figure largely in their plans for childbirth. For others, little time is spent thinking about their rights and expectations until they are asked. However, it can be very helpful to have some knowledge about the choices available to you before you make any decisions. Gaining information in good time will allow you to make informed choices about your future with your little one.

Maternity leave

Whether you have planned your pregnancy or not, it is important to make some plans for after the birth, especially if you work as your employer will need to know how much time you intend to take off.

It is common for women to return to work within six to nine months of the birth, especially if they are not used to being at home or not working. However, some women plan to take as much time off as possible or even give up work altogether for the foreseeable future.

What is maternity leave and who is entitled?

In the UK there are two types of maternity leave: ordinary maternity leave and additional maternity leave. Every worker has the right to receive 26 weeks of ordinary maternity leave regardless of the length of service to their employer, how much they earn, how many hours they are on or otherwise, as long as they give their employer the correct amount of notice. This leave can be

'Whether you have planned your pregnancy or not, it is important to make some plans for after the birth, especially if you work as your employer will need to know how much time you intend to take off.'

topped up with a further 26 weeks of additional maternity which may be taken without pay. As from October 2008, your contractual rights during these times are the same and you will also be entitled to your normal amount of annual leave on top of this leave.

Your employer will be able to tell you exactly how to go about arranging maternity leave, how to fill in the forms and who to send them to.

Maternity pay and payments

The amount of payment you receive during your time on maternity leave depends on many things, such as your salary, your duration of service to your employer and whether you have given your employer a copy of your MAT B1 certificate (this is issued by your midwife at around 20 weeks).

'While some women cope well with having time off work, others cannot get used to it and look forward to their return.'

Please seek further advice on your rights and expectations from your human resources department, Citizens Advice Bureau or the Department of Work and Pensions, as they may be able to calculate exactly how much payment you are entitled to.

If you are not working, have recently changed jobs or are self-employed, you may be entitled to a maternity allowance. You can be assessed for this by sending your MAT B1 form to your nearest Jobcentre Plus or Social Security office.

Please note that maternity leave and pay may vary as per local policy – see your employer for further information.

Returning to work

Returning to work is a subject that you have probably already spent a lot of time thinking about. While some women cope well with having time off work, others cannot get used to it and look forward to their return.

It is essential that the subject is addressed and suitable childcare options are organised. It is also important to consider whether you need to change your working circumstances, hours or shift pattern and whether this is suitable for your new situation.

If you are breastfeeding and want to continue to do so when you have returned to work, this is also an issue that needs thought. Perhaps you are going to need to express your milk during the day and store it until you return home, in which case you may need to ask your employer to install a suitable fridge in your workplace to allow for adequate and safe storage of the milk. You should also be given time when needed to perform the expressing of the milk. This should not affect your legal break entitlements.

Finding a work-life balance

Finding a work-life balance can be tricky and is often a subject that many men and women don't spend much time thinking about until they have already returned to work.

Initially, you may feel as though you will cope very well with full time work and using childcare, and for many families this works very well. For others, the demands of a busy job coupled with bringing up a child can be too much and often individual circumstances may dictate that a change is needed.

If you are looking to make changes in your work to balance it against your personal life, please make sure you have spoken at length to your partner and employer as there may be a very simple solution that can benefit both parties.

In extreme circumstances, you may feel as though you need to look for alternative employment while your family is young. There are, however, many laws now in place that aim to help those with young children, and your employer may be obliged to try and help you if they are able.

Rights for employees returning to work

It is never too early to start planning how you will fit parenthood in with your working life. If you choose to continue in your existing employment after your maternity leave, you may want to think about reducing your hours or changing your shift patterns so that you can enjoy a healthy work-life balance.

Flexible hours

Most employees have the right to request a more flexible approach to their working pattern with the exception of those in the armed forces and those who are agency workers. It may be granted to people who have a dependent or are caring for someone, so those with a newborn or young child are in a good position.

Flexible working can mean several things. It may mean that you would like to alter your contracted hours or shift pattern, explore job-sharing schemes or change your scheduled break times.

'Most employees have the right to request a more flexible approach to their working pattern with the exception of those in the armed forces and those who are agency workers.'

Your employer must give your request considerable thought and can only really reject it if it does not make good business sense. They should also explain their reasons if your requests get rejected. Even if you are not permitted to request flexible working patterns, it won't hurt to ask – your employer might find your request fits in better with their objectives than you initially thought.

Please visit www.direct.gov.uk for more information regarding your rights to flexible working.

Changing your contracted hours

Many women, especially those who work full time before they have their first child, decide that it is more suitable to return to work on fewer contracted hours than before their maternity leave. This is very common and usually quite possible.

At the earliest opportunity you should speak to either your boss or your human resources department for guidance on how to go about making this request. Your employer (with the exception of a few) is obliged to seriously consider this request and try to find ways of fitting it in with their business objectives.

Perhaps going part time will open up the opportunity of a job-sharing scheme for another potential employee, which can be beneficial to the company.

Always remember that by reducing your hours you may lose out on some benefits, such as receiving the same pension as before. Make sure you are fully informed on how reducing your hours may affect your situation before you change your contract, and seek further advice if necessary.

When your child is unwell

If you have a child under five and have worked for your current employer for at least one year, you are entitled to take up to 13 weeks of parental leave. This may not be paid leave but employers must allow this time.

The only differential is if your child is disabled, in which case you will be entitled to up to 18 weeks of leave until your child is 18-years-old.

You can also ask for time off in a child-related emergency but, again, this may not necessarily be paid leave.

Parental leave

Your parental leave may be used to spend quality time with your child, stay with them in hospital if needed or even to help find more suitable childcare arrangements. This leave will probably be unpaid and should not affect your rights when you return to work.

Attending medical appointments

As a pregnant woman you are entitled to take time off to attend medical appointments and antenatal care during your pregnancy. You are also entitled to take time off to have the baby and afterwards. Your employer, however, does not necessarily have to pay you while you are not working.

After you have had the baby, you have no actual rights to attend doctor's appointments and the like, though most employers are quite flexible. You do, however, have the right to unpaid time off if your child is unwell.

Your financial rights

Having a child can be very expensive, especially if it is your first and you have no baby-related items already stored from a previous child. Fortunately, you may be able to top up your income or savings with a little extra help.

'If you have a child under five and have worked for your current employer for at least one year, you are entitled to take up to 13 weeks of parental leave.'

Child Benefit

Child Benefit is a payment given to parents to help with the costs of bringing up a child. Even better is the fact that it is tax free and you are entitled to it.

If your child is under 16 and you contribute financially to their upbringing, you can receive Child Benefit.

As from January 2009, your payment will be £20 a week for your first child, with a further £12.55 a week for subsequent children until they are 16 (slightly older if they are in further education).

The payment can be paid directly into your bank usually monthly, though weekly payments can be arranged if you contact the Child Benefit office.

'If your child is under 16 and you contribute financially to their upbringing, you can receive Child Benefit.'

Tax Credit

Tax Credits are payments made to those who qualify for help with the costs of bringing up a child.

The system, however, is quite complicated and the criteria and payments made are dependent on your individual circumstances. They can be affected by your partner's wage, the hours you work and your individual salary.

It is advised that you visit www.direct.gov.uk or contact the Tax Credit Helpline (0845 300 3909) for more information or to apply for Tax Credit. As you are expecting your first child, the chances are that you will be entitled to some additional funds.

Help with childcare costs

If you are working and are expecting to return to work once you have had your baby and finished your maternity leave, you may be worried about the costs of childcare and how you will manage financially. However, don't panic until you have found out whether you are entitled to help with childcare costs.

Many working parents pay for childcare and a good percentage of these receive financial help with the costs. Depending on your individual circumstances, salary and expected costs, your case will be assessed and your entitlements will be calculated, giving you a greater opportunity to work and be a parent.

Telephone the Tax Credit Helpline on 0845 300 3909, speak to an adviser and ask whether you will qualify for any help towards childcare costs when you return to work.

It is likely, however, that you will only receive a rough estimate until your childcare costs have been verified (and you've applied for them) and it's been checked that the childcare you have arranged is being carried out by a qualified and registered provider (not by a friend or relative).

Child Trust Funds

Parents of children born after September 2002 are now entitled to a small amount of money that will help secure the child's future. This is called a Child Trust Fund and is granted after application.

To some degree, parents are allowed to make a choice as to where the money should be saved, with the aim of it growing into a fairly good sized nest-egg when the child turns 18.

What are Child Trust Funds?

Child Trust Funds are one-off payments given to new parents. They can either be put into a savings account or invested (via an organised business, normally a bank) in stocks and shares.

The parents can select what they do with the money (which comes in a voucher form) and when the decision has been made and the voucher sent, the account cannot be withdrawn from by anyone except the child (however, they cannot acces it until they are 18).

'Many working parents pay for childcare and a good percentage of these receive financial help with the costs.'

It is possible that the account can be added to and many parents choose to arrange a small amount to be transferred to the fund each month, allowing it to grow quite considerably in 18 years.

Please speak to an independent financial adviser, your local bank or visit www.childtrustfund.gov.uk for more information and advice about this subject.

Summing Up

Looking after your physical and mental health is the most important thing during pregnancy, but it can help to make sure you are organised after the birth as well. Ensuring your employer is aware of your plans is vital in relieving many of the pressures facing working parents.

As a pregnant woman you will find that you are fairly well protected in the workplace both before and after the birth. You will be entitled to several payments and rights when you have the baby and after returning to work.

It is possible that your employer may not be aware of all your rights and entitlements, especially if you work in a male dominated environmet. Carrying out your own research into these areas may benefit you if you can provide your boss with all the facts surrounding your condition and parenthood.

Chapter Eleven

The Expectant Father or Partner

It is not just the pregnant woman who is involved in the pregnancy, you, as her partner (and/or father of the child), should have a great deal of involvement too. After all, this is your child and you have rights, fears and expectations, and are about to start a new chapter in life.

The subject of pregnancy is still invariably centred on the mum-to-be and the developing child, as it should be, but there are now many areas and agencies that realise the vital role that fathers and partners play in the whole process. It is now recognised that they should not be excluded or neglected during this time.

Studies have proved that in safe home environments, where the father of the child is around, women have less stressful pregnancies. It is also recognised that the child has a better bond with the father after the birth if they are actively involved in the child rearing process. Therefore, it is important to make sure that you are included both in the pregnancy and the childcare and parenting after the birth.

'From discovering the pregnancy to making up feeds, there are thousands of ways you can be actively involved and enjoy being a parent from the start.'

Supporting your partner

There are many ways in which you can be a support to your partner during the pregnancy and childbirth process, and this does not simply mean running and fetching endless cups of tea!

From discovering the pregnancy to making up feeds, there are thousands of ways you can be actively involved and enjoy being a parent from the start.

Discovering the pregnancy

Finding out your partner is pregnant can be a shock, especially if you were not planning for a child. It normally causes feelings of elation followed by uncertainty and wonder as to whether you are ready to take on this responsibility. In a few cases, it can cause the partner to feel as though they want to take time out and absorb the information before they respond. Each reaction is natural – it is how you manage these emotions that counts.

Your partner will have suspected she was pregnant in the first instance in order to warrant taking a test. Your response cannot be predicted but she will have pondered about your reaction.

The best result is when both parties are ecstatic with the pregnancy. They can celebrate the news together and allow themselves to revel in it for a while before they tell others. If, however, you are unsure of how you feel, spend some thinking it over before you reveal your feelings to your partner. Remember, these are memories you will carry with you for the rest of your life, so be sure of how you feel before you react. Similarly, if your partner suspects she is pregnant, or you have been actively trying, maybe you could go out together and select a pregnancy test or two to take as a couple.

It is natural to feel unsure as to whether you are ready to be a parent, or if you will be a good parent, and the chances are your partner will be having exactly the same doubts. These are parts of the pregnancy that can be explored together and may even bring you closer, demonstrating that because you are having these thoughts and discussing them with each other, you are indeed ready and mature enough to be parents.

Feeling left out

As your partner gets used to having a dependent and begins to learn how to be a parent, it is likely that you may feel a bit left out. All of a sudden you have gone from being your partner's priority to being second on the list, and this can be an unusual feeling.

The best way to handle this situation is to become the main support mechanism to your partner. She will be tired (as you may be too) and will need help with the little one. After all, you are both parents to the baby.

Use the time to find your own independence and become an example to the child by assuming some of the other roles around the house. You could decide to do all the cooking or organise the dirty laundry. You could even take charge of the baby sometimes, showing your partner you are capable too.

Try not to let yourself become jealous of your son or daughter as this is highly unproductive and will only serve to become a problem in the future. Your new child is a tiny baby and needs you as much as its mother, so you need to be a parent too, not a rival for your partner's affection.

In the first few months of pregnancy

The first few months of pregnancy can be quite difficult for the expectant father or partner of the pregnant woman. Not only have you just received the news that you are to become a parent, but you will have a lot of emotions to deal with from both yourself and your partner.

Women are notoriously hormonal in the first few months of pregnancy and this can bring many sudden changes of mood and circumstance. You may find that your partner is irritable and snappy, and unfortunately this is just a normal part of pregnancy, so try not to let it get you down too much. Try to understand that it is part of the process and something that many expectant parents experience.

Patience is vital during the first few weeks and being supportive is essential in remaining a strong and stable couple. Offering this support may include taking on more responsibility around the home, getting used to your partner's food fads and giving her space when she needs it.

You may feel extremely protective of your partner and fall into the trap of constantly telling her to take it easy or put her feet up, and for some women this is lovely, while others find it stifling and become annoyed. Remember that she may not feel pregnant at all in the first few months and will carry on as before; you will need to take your cue from her actions and reactions.

'As your partner gets used to having a dependent and begins to learn how to be a parent, it is likely that you may feel a bit left out.'

It is also extremely pro-active to use this time to make your own lifestyle healthier; your partner will be drinking little or no alcohol for the foreseeable future, so you could choose to do this too. Why not both make more of an effort to get more exercise by making time for walks when you can? You could even start planning any changes you may need to make in your home.

Overall, this should be an exciting time and can provide many opportunities for planning and participating in activities together. Embrace it while you can.

Dealing with your own emotions

It is not just your partner's emotions that will be significantly affected by the pregnancy and what having a child can mean. You are likely to question your own capabilities as a parent (as your own parents probably did) and you may feel scared. For many people (especially men), this is an unfamiliar emotion and can take some adjustment.

'You are likely to question your own capabilities as a parent... and you may feel scared.'

Above all, you should remember that you are not alone. Although the focal point of the pregnancy is on your partner and the baby, there are services around that can offer support to the expectant father or partner, and many of the available websites contain whole sections aimed specifically at dads-to-be. Many of them also include forums so you can discuss your feelings and experiences with other dads and partners in the same position as yourself.

Fears and expectancies

Being scared is a common part of being an expectant father. You may be frightened of your own performance and parenting abilities, or scared that something may go wrong and that you will be left bereaved or unable to cope. You might worry whether you can cope with a crying baby and the responsibility and patience that being a parent requires.

For most, these fears are absolved as soon as the baby lets out the first cry and all toes and fingers are present and correct. For others who do face challenges, they take these in their stride and accept them as part of being a parent, through the bad times and the good.

You would be pretty unique if you didn't have fears and anxieties at all.

Supporting through labour

There are many ways you can be a support through the labour: from fetching drinks and offering reassurance to giving massages and mopping her brow.

Your role during this time is fairly undefined and will be unique – each birth is individual and can't really be planned to the last detail.

Perhaps your partner has some specific requests that involve you or maybe you can offer support by making sure all her requests are carried out. Even if things don't go exactly to plan, you will probably find the whole experience turns out fine in the end.

The first few weeks

In the first few weeks you may find that your partner is reluctant to let you do anything with the baby or has no time for you. This is totally normal and is now the time for you to prove to her that you can do housework and cook, and also that you want to be involved with the baby. Make sure you take your turn feeding and bathing the baby but also that you know how to do it; before leaving the hospital, your wife or partner will have been taught how to do all of these things.

Paternity leave

As you have just become a father, you are now equally responsible for the upbringing and keep of your child. If you are employed, you are entitled to take some paternity leave.

What is paternity leave?

Paternity leave is a form of authorised absence from work that allows you to spend time at home with your partner, getting to know your baby and supporting your new family after the birth.

Who is entitled to paternity leave?

The right to paternity leave depends on what sort of employment you are currently undertaking. If you are a contracted employee, you will probably be entitled to take some paternity leave with pay as long as you have been employed for at least 26 weeks from the last day of the 15th week before the baby was due.

If, however, you are a casual worker, do not have a contract, work within an agency or otherwise, you may be able to take some leave but you are not likely to receive any pay for this period.

'As you have just become a father, you are now equally responsible for the upbringing and keep of your child. If you are employed, you are entitled to take some paternity leave.'

Paternity leave is currently two weeks which can be taken at any time between the birth of the child and 56 days after delivery. The leave must be taken consecutively and weeks cannot be split. Paternity leave is usually paid if you earn £90 or more per week before tax.

Applying for paternity leave

To find out if you qualify for paternity leave, please go to www.direct.gov.uk for more information or speak to your human resources department. They will be able to tell you if you qualify for full pay on your leave and how to make your application.

Returning to work

Returning to work after the birth of your child may make you feel uncomfortable as you have just established a bond with your child; this is especially hard if your partner is still at home because you may feel excluded. Likewise, it may be a big relief to go back to work as your timetable is likely to have turned fairly abnormal, and you may feel you could benefit from finding a normal routine again.

Unfortunately, returning to work is a fact of life for most and is something that cannot be avoided. However, it can help to make sure you have set some definite rules with your partner before you return.

Discuss with your partner what role you are going to play in the life of your child and make sure you are both happy with the tasks you will carry out. For example, it may help if you offer to do the baby's bath when you get in or give him or her a bottle before bedtime so that you have a routine with them.

Achieving a work-life balance

Finding a work-life balance can be difficult and sometimes the pressure to achieve a suitable balance can be very upsetting.

If you feel as though you would like to amend your working life to suit your personal life more, try speaking to your employer and see if it would be possible to alter your shift pattern or make changes elsewhere that open up opportunities to spend more time at home.

As the child ages and your partner returns to work, deciding who can do the nursery runs, followed later by school drop-offs and pick-ups, can take an awful lot of planning. It is essential that you address these issues early on.

Worrying about the birth

Worrying about the birth is totally normal; you will probably be frightened for both your partner and the baby. Talk to your partner about your fears and decide what role you are going to play in the labour and what plans you can make.

Will I cope?

When the subject of pregnancy or birth is discussed in a general way, many men are quite specific about whether they think they will be able to cope with it or not. However, in reality, they probably won't be able to say for sure until they are actually expecting a baby themselves. Many men who felt that they wouldn't want to witness the birth actually end up saying that they wouldn't have missed it for the world, while others who thought they'd take it all in their stride suddenly couldn't cope with seeing their partner in so much pain and waited outside.

Worrying about what you will do can be exhausting, so it is probably best to discuss your fears with your partner, finding out what her wishes are and whether she wants anyone else to accompany her throughout the delivery.

It is also highly beneficial to try and attend the antenatal classes with your partner, as these can be very useful for the expectant dad. They help to answer all of your questions and take away some of the mystery and wonderment of pregnancy and childbirth. Attending these classes can really help to ease some of your fears as well.

Helping your partner through labour can be a long and arduous process and it can be emotionally and physically exhausting for you too, so make sure you are taking some time out to have a drink, a snack and to stretch your legs. You are no good to your partner if you are not well yourself!

I don't want to see the person I love in such pain

Nobody wants to see someone they love in pain and it can be very difficult to watch your partner go through labour.

The midwife can be very useful for finding out more information regarding pain relief and you may want to discuss your fears with her, either before the labour or when you are at the hospital. You will be far more use to your partner if you are prepared than if you haven't done any groundwork and are distressed during the birth.

I'm squeamish

Worrying about what you will see and how you will cope during the birth is something that bothers many birthing partners and expectant parents.

The chances are you will be so wrapped up in the miracle that you are part of, you will forget about your fears, allowing awe and excitement to take over.

However, if you are particularly worried about fainting, feeling unwell or being more of a hindrance than a help, you should discuss your concerns with the mother-to-be and also the midwife. Perhaps you could stay towards your

'Helping your partner through labour can be a long and arduous process and it can be emotionally and physically exhausting for you too, so make sure you are taking some time out to have a drink, a snack and to stretch your legs.'

partner's head during the entire delivery or would feel better if you just waited outside? If this is the case, you should make sure that there is someone else who can be your partner's birthing support.

What if something goes wrong?

This fear does not only affect you but will be going through the mind of your partner as well. Even though people have been having babies forever, there is still the potential for things to go wrong either late in pregnancy or during the birth. The best solution to this is to make sure you both lead healthy lifestyles in preparation of the pregnancy and during the pregnancy itself.

It is also essential to attend all appointments and undergo all the tests that your doctor or midwife advises you to take. This enables any potential problems to be spotted early and treatment can be planned.

Worrying that something bad will happen to your baby or your partner during the birth is something that all expectant fathers and partners go through and, unfortunately, there may be nothing you can do to ease these fears entirely. Medical research and equipment has totally changed the dangers involved with childbirth and there are far fewer complications these days than there were even 50 years ago, so some comfort can be taken from this.

My partner doesn't want me at the birth

Although it happens less these days, there are still some circumstances when your partner may not want you to be with them during the birth. This may be because of personal or cultural reasons, because she fears you will not cope with it very well or because she doesn't want you to see her 'like that'. For the most part, you must respect her wishes, and some men are actually relieved that they don't need to attend and are satisfied with waiting outside the delivery room. However, if you do want to attend, it is important to discuss your partner's reasons before labour begins and understand why she feels like this. You never know, you may find that she is fearful of you finding her less attractive or feels she is 'letting you off the hook' by making the decision for you.

Your relationship

It is a fact of life for most couples that their lifestyle will alter after the arrival of their first child, but there is also the chance that your relationship may be temporarily affected. This can happen for a number of reasons but there are ways of making sure you continue to communicate and spend quality time together.

Finding time for each other

'Try and make sure you have at least half an hour each evening when the baby is asleep without the television being on, so that you can talk and enjoy each other's company for a while.'

In the first few weeks your baby will dictate your timetable and you may find that you are taking it in turns to sleep. Making the effort to spend even a few minutes alone (or just together) can be a real help in keeping your relationship solid.

Try and make sure you have at least half an hour each evening when the baby is asleep without the television being on, so that you can talk and enjoy each other's company for a while. Perhaps you could make the extra effort and cook a nice meal once or twice a week and enjoy eating together. You may have to attend to the baby once or twice but the effort will be appreciated and it will help keep the romance alive.

Communication

Good communication is an essential element of child rearing. It is vital that you communicate effectively when dealing with relationship problems, childcare issues and even the general running of the home.

Remember that tiredness can make people very irritable and this can mean a small disagreement soon leads to a full-scale argument. During this time, try and have a little more patience with each other and make sure that you spend some time together every day, doing something you enjoy or talking.

Feeling left out with a newborn

Many new dads feel as though they are being left out because their partner has a new priority. However, this feeling will pass.

The relationship and feelings your partner has for you are very different from those for her child. When a baby is very young, they are solely dependent on their parents, so yes, you may have to take a back seat for a while.

However, try to remember that this is your baby too and you can shoulder some of the day to day jobs and duties, making the family dynamic, more equal and well balanced.

Your partner's changing body

Your partner's body after childbirth will probably have changed dramatically from before she was pregnant. For some, this is permanent, while others find they return to their previous figure quite quickly.

All of the marks, lines and weight gain are part of the natural process of pregnancy and childbirth and, unfortunately, come as part of the package!

The worst thing to do would be to make a huge issue out of it and make your partner feel even more self-conscious. This may cause her to feel less attractive and less inclined to resume a physical relationship.

Try and bolster her confidence with some nice comments and try to raise her self-esteem.

Sex after the birth

Your partner's body has just been through a very demanding experience and it is no wonder that she may not be in the mood for a few months after the birth. It may be that she is still suffering some of the after effects of giving birth or is simply too tired or frightened to have sex; these issues are all normal. Be patient, make sure she knows you understand and try to find other ways of being close to each other instead. Massage, talking, rubbing her feet, running her a bath or even a simple cuddle will reassure her that you still find her attractive, but don't be tempted to push the subject too much or it may become a big issue.

If you are concerned you could just ask her to let you know when she is ready to resume a physical relationship, relieving some of the pressure.

Some women, however, find that they are feeling very sexual shortly after the birth, though penetration should be avoided for at least six weeks so that everything can return to normal. But please remember that women are at their most fertile after giving birth, so it is essential that you use a suitable form of contraception. Also remember that the pregnancy may have altered your partner's body slightly, so try and keep any observations to yourself.

Bonding with your child

Many fathers worry about whether they will bond with their baby in the same way as their partner beacuse they haven't experienced the pregnancy in the same way. These feelings are totally natural and there are many things you can do to make sure you bond with your child.

Bonding with your child before it is born

Before your baby is born, you can feel it move by placing your hand over the bump during an active time. You can also sing and talk to your partner's bump so that the baby can hear your voice and learn to recognise it. You may also want to attend all appointments and support your partner by using massage or changing your own diet to suit that of a pregnant woman to get the most out of the experience.

Babies that breastfeed

If your partner is planning to breastfeed, you can still find magical times for bonding with your child. Why don't you suggest that you do all the baby baths for the first few months? This way, your baby knows that this is their alone time with you and will look forward to it.

You may also want to discuss the notion of expressing breast milk, which is particularly good for very demanding babies or those who do not fully empty the breast of its milk. This means your baby will get all the benefits of breast milk but has the chance of being fed by you or another friend or family member.

'Make sure you know what is happening to your partner and child during the pregnancy by doing your own reading and asking any questions you feel you need to.'

Summing Up

During a pregnancy the mother-to-be and the developing baby are the most important considerations and will be closely monitored and assessed. However, your needs are important too and sometimes 'dad' can feel a little bit out of the loop.

Make sure you know what is happening to your partner and child during the pregnancy by doing your own reading and asking any questions you feel you need to.

Always remember that this is your child too. You will be an equal in the parenting stakes and may need to be assertive to make sure you are heard.

If you are feeling vulnerable, left out or are worrying about the birth, why not involve yourself with the pregnancy more and go to some antenatal classes? You could even join a fathers' group. This way, you can discuss your issues openly in a like-minded group of other dads.

Being a dad is important and you are likely to be the person who offers the most support and assistance during the pregnancy and birth, so be open with your partner and allow her to guide you through the experience.

Help List

Askbaby.com

Askbaby.com, Fleet House, 8-12 New Bridge Street, London, EC4V 6AL
contact@askbaby.com
www.askbaby.com
Website giving information and advice on conception, pregnancy and childbirth.

Association of Breastfeeding Mothers

ABM, PO Box 207, Bridgwater, Somerset, TA6 7YT
Tel: 08444 122949 (helpline)
counselling@abm.me.uk
www.abm.me.uk
A charity founded by mothers for mothers to provide accurate information on breastfeeding.

Babyandpregnancy.co.uk

www.babyandpregnancy.co.uk
Website including articles on all aspects of pregnancy and birth. You can join and receive newsletters or even send in your own stories.

Babycentre

www.babycentre.co.uk
This website offers a comprehensive guide to the entire pregnancy, with detailed articles on the subject along with baby name suggestions, calculators and calendars. There are also sections for expectant fathers and partners and a facility to join forums, start blogs and share stories and photos.

Babyworld

Mongewell Park Farm, Wallingford Road, Wallingford, Oxon, OX10 8DY
www.babyworld.co.uk
This site is a UK-based network that is full of information on fertility, pregnancy and parenting. It offers professional advice, support from other parents, shopping ideas, discounts, competitions and much more. You should be able to find out all the information you need.

Bounty

www.bounty.com
Online club for mums-to-be and new mums, offering news, advice and competitions.

Breastfedbabies.org

Health Promotion Agency, 18 Ormeau Avenue, Belfast, BT2 8HS
Tel: 02890 311611 (8.45am-5pm, Monday to Thursday, 8.45am-4.30pm, Friday.)
info@breastfedbabies.org
www.breastfedbabies.org
A website run by the Health Promotion Agency of Northern Ireland, providing information on breastfeeding and its benefits. It also gives details of local support groups.

Breastfeeding Network

PO Box 11126, Paisley, PA2 8YB
Tel: 08444 124664 (supportline)
breastfeedingnetwork@googlemail.com
www.breastfeedingnetwork.org.uk
The Breastfeeding Network provides information, advice and support on all aspects of breastfeeding. It also gives details of local centres.

Care Confidential

Clarendon House, 9-11 Church Street, Basingstoke, RG21 7QG
Tel: 0800 028 2228 (helpline)
careconfidential@care.org.uk
www.careconfidential.com
This service offers a confidential advisory telephone service for those wanting to discuss private and delicate issues in a totally confidential setting. If your pregnancy was unplanned or was the result of a rape or sexual assault, you can discuss all your emotions and options. Whatever your needs, there will always be someone you can talk to privately and securely.

Child Trust Funds

Child Trust Funds Office, Waterview Park, Mandarin Way, Washington, NE38 8QG
Tel: 0845 3021470 (helpline 8am-8pm)
0845 3021489 (helpline for Welsh speakers 8.30am-5pm, Monday to Friday.)
www.childtrustfund.gov.uk
A website for the office of long term savings and investment accounts for children, introduced by the government.

Citizens Advice Bureau

Myddelten House, 115-123 Pentonville Road, London, N1 9LZ
www.citizensadvice.org.uk
CAB is a charity with offices all over the country. They offer free information, advice and help with resolving financial and other problems.

Department of Work and Pensions

Caxton House, Tothill Street, London, SW1H 9DA
www.dwp.gov.uk
Government organisation dealing with all matters related to employment.
See their website for details of different departments and contact details for local offices.

DirectGov

www.direct.gov.uk
A website offering details on all government departments and agencies, including information on parental benefits.

Fertility Expert

www.fertilityexpert.co.uk
This site offers a plethora of information on all aspects of fertility, offering advice on how to achieve pregnancy, getting fertility help and the emotional aspects surrounding the subject.

For Parents By Parents

www.forparentsbyparents.com
Information and advice by parents for expectant parents and parents of children up to the age of five.

Mama (Meet a Mum Association)

Tel: 0845 1203746 (helpline 7pm-10pm, Monday to Friday)
www.mama.co.uk
MAMA is a charity created to help mothers who feel depressed and isolated after giving birth. The website gives details of local groups and contacts.

Maternity Action

The Grayston Centre, 28 Charles Square, London, N1 6HT
Tel: 020 73244740
www.maternityaction.org.uk
This website offers a mine of information regarding the rights and legal issues surrounding pregnancy and maternity issues. It aims to provide advice, support and demonstration of best practice to pregnant women, their family and their place of employment.

National Childbirth Trust (NCT)

Alexandra House, Oldham Terrace, London, W3 6NH
Tel: 0300 3300772 (pregnancy and birth line)
0300 3300771 (breastfeeding line)
0300 3300770 (enquiries line)
www.nctpregnancyandbabycare.com
One of the largest charities for parents, the NCT website gives details of support groups throughout the country and information to parents during and after pregnancy.

Netmums

124 Mildred Avenue, Watford, Herts, WD18 7DX
contactus@netmums.com
www.netmums.com
This site is excellent for finding local networks of new, experienced and expectant mums, aiming to put local people in touch with each other. There are forums, coffee shops and professional guidance for pregnancy and parenting issues. Advice is also provided on just about every aspect of parenting, including the difficulties that may be faced and unusual circumstances.

Pampers

Tel: 0800 3283281
www.pampers.co.uk
Offering a week-by-week guide to pregnancy, this household name provides a good source of information on pregnancy and information about children of a pre-school age.

Parentline Plus

520 Highgate Studios, 53-79 Highgate Road, Kentish Town, London, NW5 1TL
Tel: 0808 8002222 (helpline)
020 7284 5500 (general information)
www.parentlineplus.org.uk
Parentline Plus is a national charity working for and with parents. It offers information, support and links to other useful services.

Raising Kids

RaisingKids.co.uk, Disney Interactive Media Group, 3 Queen Caroline Street, London, W6 9PE
Tel: 020 8222 3923
feedback@raisingkids.co.uk
www.raisingkids.co.uk
A website founded by a parenting expert, Raising Kids gives advice, information and tips from conception right through to the teenage years.

Single Parent Action Network

Millpond, Baptist Street, Easton, Bristol, B25 0YW
Tel: 0117 9514231
www.singleparents.org.uk
This group is a useful organisation representing single parents all over the UK. They provide plenty of information on single parent issues, giving people the tools and knowledge to make significant changes for single parents in their own area of the UK.

Single Parents

www.onespace.org.uk
An online resource for single parents in the UK. Make friends, ask an expert for advice or simply browse the site at your leisure. With resources like this, you won't be alone for long.

The Twins and Multiple Birth Association (TAMBA)

2 The Willows, Gardner Road, Guilford, GU1 4PG
Tel: 0800 1380509 (helpline)
www.tamba.org.uk
Offering support to parents of multiples in general, this is a resource for information, latest news and developments.

Twins Club

PO Box 9494, Redditch, Worcs, B98 8PQ
www.twinsclub.co.uk
If you need extra support during your multiple pregnancy or raising your children, then this site is definitely worth a look. Filled with ideas and support for those parenting twins or more, it includes sections advertising items for sale, deatils of local groups in the UK and even a chatroom.

Need - 2 - Know

Available Titles Include ...

Allergies A Parent's Guide
ISBN 978-1-86144-064-8 £8.99

Autism A Parent's Guide
ISBN 978-1-86144-069-3 £8.99

Drugs A Parent's Guide
ISBN 978-1-86144-043-3 £8.99

Dyslexia and Other Learning Difficulties
A Parent's Guide ISBN 978-1-86144-042-6 £8.99

Bullying A Parent's Guide
ISBN 978-1-86144-044-0 £8.99

Epilepsy The Essential Guide
ISBN 978-1-86144-063-1 £8.99

Teenage Pregnancy The Essential Guide
ISBN 978-1-86144-046-4 £8.99

Gap Years The Essential Guide
ISBN 978-1-86144-079-2 £8.99

How to Pass Exams A Parent's Guide
ISBN 978-1-86144-047-1 £8.99

Child Obesity A Parent's Guide
ISBN 978-1-86144-049-5 £8.99

Applying to University The Essential Guide
ISBN 978-1-86144-052-5 £8.99

ADHD The Essential Guide
ISBN 978-1-86144-060-0 £8.99

Student Cookbook - Healthy Eating The Essential Guide
ISBN 978-1-86144-061-7 £8.99

Stress The Essential Guide
ISBN 978-1-86144-054-9 £8.99

Adoption and Fostering A Parent's Guide
ISBN 978-1-86144-056-3 £8.99

Special Educational Needs A Parent's Guide
ISBN 978-1-86144-057-0 £8.99

The Pill An Essential Guide
ISBN 978-1-86144-058-7 £8.99

University A Survival Guide
ISBN 978-1-86144-072-3 £8.99

Diabetes The Essential Guide
ISBN 978-1-86144-059-4 £8.99

View the full range at **www.need2knowbooks.co.uk**. To order our titles, call **01733 898103**, email **sales@n2kbooks.com** or visit the website.

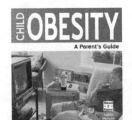
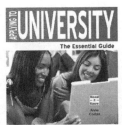
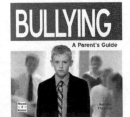
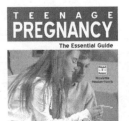
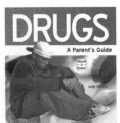

Need - 2 - Know, Remus House, Coltsfoot Drive, Peterborough, PE2 9JX